THE
DUKAN
DIET

THE
DUKAN
DIET

2 Steps to Lose the Weight,
2 Steps to Keep It Off
Forever

Dr. Pierre Dukan

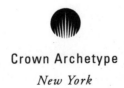

Crown Archetype
New York

Originally published in paperback in France as *Je Ne Sais Pas Maigrir* by
Flammarion, an imprint of the Flammarion Groupe, Paris, 2000.
This English translation was originally published in paperback in slightly
different form in Great Britain by Hodder & Stoughton, an Hachette UK
company, London, in 2010.

Library of Congress Cataloging-in-Publication Data
Dukan, Pierre, doctor.
The Dukan diet : 2 steps to lose the weight, 2 steps to keep it off forever /
Pierre Dukan.
    p. cm.
    1. Reducing diets—Popular works.   2. Weight loss—Popular
works.   I. Title.
    RM222.2.D74   2011
613.2'5—dc22
2010045601

ISBN 978-0-307-88796-2
eISBN 978-0-307-88797-9

PRINTED IN THE UNITED STATES OF AMERICA

Jacket design by Jean Traina

20 19

For Sacha and Maya,

for Maya and Sacha,

my two children,

for the second life they have offered me,

in return for the gift of life I have given to them.

To Christine, my wife,

without whom this endeavor

could never have even been imagined.

To Sylvia and Maurice,

who still speak through me.

CONTENTS

RECIPES AND MENUS

THE
DUKAN
DIET

On April 12, 1945, the day that President Roosevelt died, my brother was born. My family, which is Jewish, named him Franklin in recognition of what this great president did to liberate Europe, France, and the French people. My father realized that without America's intervention, my brother would never have been born or been able to bear this first name.

For the rest of his life, my father continued to admire and feel great affection for the American nation. Although in the second half of the twentieth century there was no shortage of tension and fraternal quarreling between our two countries, my father held steadfast to his creed: "Never forget that the Americans saved us," he would say. "We are indebted to them. If one day you find yourself in a situation where you can show them our gratitude, do this with all your heart."

As I write this note for the American edition, I am moved to think of my father, because I feel that in bringing this book to America, I am carrying out his wish. I come to you and also your Canadian neighbors with a weight loss method to which I have devoted thirty-five years of my life and which has been tried and tested in almost every corner of the world.

I am a medical doctor in the field of nutrition. Very early on in my professional career I specialized in fighting against weight problems, a field in which contemporary medicine had failed to make any headway. Inspired by one of my patients, I started specializing in treating weight problems through personal consultations. Very quickly I devised my own tools and a diet that suited my patients' psychology, as well as their metabolism—a diet that was much more successful for them than the low-calorie diets prevalent at that time. Seeing how effective this plan was and how it produced far better results, I soon felt the need to try to help a wider public. When I was sure that my four-phase weight loss method had shown proven results, I turned it into a book dedicated to the general public as well as to my medical peers in France.

In the past ten years, this book has become a publishing phenomenon, selling 2 million copies in France, where it has been at the top of the best-seller list since 2006. The Dukan Diet then became an Internet phenomenon as a community of 10 million men and women sprang up, exchanging their ideas on five hundred websites, forums, and blogs dedicated to my method. At the same time, this diet was crossing borders and becoming established in over thirty countries, including England, Korea, Brazil, and Poland, and in doing so it has proved its universal appeal.

I am not giving you this background out of immodesty but rather to offer evidence of the effectiveness of this diet and the enthusiasm with which it has been received internationally. To be honest, the scale of this worldwide movement and the immense wealth of friendship, kindness, and emotional closeness that it has set in motion has been a tremendous gift to me—and an equally tremendous surprise.

Offering you the Dukan Diet is both my greatest challenge and my greatest risk. In recent years, several opportunities arose to get this book published in North America and to see my method do battle with North America's weight problems. I chose instead to wait, for in truth the North American audience scared me somewhat. To me North America represents the ultimate test of this diet, and I wanted to take this challenge on when I had the very best chance of succeeding.

When everything seemed just right and I had found my publisher, I began further research to tailor my diet for a North American audience. I chair an international association of nutritionists, and I asked its American members for help, for I needed to grasp the deep and personal nature of what it is to be overweight in America.

I gained even greater reassurance from seeing Americans and Canadians buy my books on Amazon UK and from the number of North

American users on the British coaching website for the diet. I carefully followed the progress of these North American users. I conversed with them in chat sessions, and I read their reports, their questions, their testimonials, and their recipe suggestions. I also immersed myself in the American way of life. I spent hours in American supermarkets and restaurants, I read American magazines, I listened to American TV programs, and I took part in discussions on American blogs and forums.

All my American research led me to two conflicting conclusions.

First, the problem of being overweight appeared to me more difficult in America than anywhere else because Americans are at the forefront of technological progress and also at the forefront of one of present-day civilization's major afflictions—being overweight. Each year in the United States, every second patent aims to cut down physical effort and to save time and in so doing encourages stress and a sedentary lifestyle. America's consumer society has brought riches and power, but also weight problems for which you are paying the highest price: 72 million Americans are obese, and in Canada the number is 5.5 million, their lives shortened daily by the excess weight they carry.

While attending a conference in Houston, I had the opportunity of meeting one of the most eminent public relations professionals in North America. We talked about weight problems and how they are such a blight in our world. He knew about my method, about how it had developed and spread, and about my plans to bring it to North America. "Nowadays, for a method to get established on North American soil, however well it works, its promoters will need to invest millions of dollars in public relations and marketing," he said. "The market for weight loss programs is saturated; there are new offers each year. If a program is new, well presented, and makes people dream, the results don't really matter." I shuddered at his words because I knew he believed what he was saying.

On the other hand, I saw the problem from a different angle. Yes, the North American cultural, economic, and political environment contributes to the escalation of weight problems. But the second conclusion I reached from my North American research was that in each North American citizen there is a human being who longs to respect the essential relationship between a healthy body and a healthy mind. I realize that most Americans and Canadians would like to lose weight but that a great many have given up on the idea because, having already tried dieting so many times in vain, they no longer believe in the hope of a real solution.

Faced with all these obstacles, I could have become disheartened about bringing this diet to the United States and Canada, but I know that of all the nations in the world, these two are the ones to which I can give the most and to which I want to give the most. Here there are lives to be saved, health and well-being to be restored. And I know in my heart of hearts that I have the means and a method that can succeed in doing this.

I know that North Americans become fired up by causes and challenges. I am setting you a cause and a challenge equal to your stature. Take this method, make it your own, and show the world how to reverse the pattern of excess weight and obesity.

Weight problems are proof of our growing difficulty in adapting to our civilization's afflictions. If you are trying to eat more healthfully, it is almost always possible to find what you are looking for, but at the same time it is very difficult not to succumb to the less healthy choices being offered to you.

For example, I am in a supermarket and am looking for a jar of pickles. But reading the label, I discover that these pickles contain sugar. So do many canned vegetables and ready-made meals. Indeed, sugar is found in a great many processed products when there is no particular reason at all for it to be there. The situation is the same with fats.

The same products without added fats and sugar exist, but you are going to have to search them out. You are going to have to scrutinize labels so that you pick the right products for your health. I am asking you to make this effort. If you want to tackle your weight problem, you have to know what you are eating.

Sometimes sugar and fats are found naturally in food. There is a lot of fat in salmon. Sugar is found in the form of lactose in yogurt and dairy products, and in the form of fructose in fruit. However, the sugar added to pickles or canned vegetables, or the fat added to some breads is neither natural nor useful. These sugars and fats seem necessary to us only because we have become used to eating them. Nowadays, added sugar and fats have become marketing tools. They are messages for our senses that are infinitely more powerful than any advertisement. They operate on our pleasure responses and condition the circuits in our brain that govern attachment and addiction.

Legislation in America and Canada requires strict food labeling for consumer protection, so learn how to make the most use of it. It just takes a few minutes to understand how to decipher any label. You will then discover, for example, that there are indeed sugar-free pickles, sugar-free canned vegetables, and sugar-free mustards out there.

My dear friends, today I am reaching out to you with the certainty that I can help you put an end to the inevitability of weight problems in North America. Now let this mutual journey begin!

—Dr. Pierre Dukan

Preface: A Decisive Encounter, or the Man Who Only Liked Meat

When I was a very young doctor, I was practicing general medicine in the Montparnasse area in Paris while also specializing in neurology for paraplegic children in Garches, just outside the capital. At that time, one of my patients was an obese, jovial, and tremendously cultivated publisher whom I treated regularly for a very trying case of asthma. One day he came to see me, and once he was seated comfortably in an armchair that creaked under his weight, he said, "Doctor, I have always been satisfied with your treatment. I trust you, and I've come to see you today because I want you to make me lose weight."

In those days, all I knew about nutrition and obesity was what my teachers had passed on at medical school, which amounted to simply suggesting low-calorie diets and miniature-sized meals so tiny that any obese person would laugh and run a mile in the opposite direction. For big eaters, the very idea of having to ration their happiness is preposterous.

I declined, stuttering under the pretext that I knew nothing of the subtleties of weight loss.

"What are you talking about? I have seen every specialist in Paris, every one of whom put me on a starvation diet. Since my teens I've lost over seven hundred pounds, and I've put it all back on again. I have to admit that I've never been deeply motivated and, without realizing it, my wife has done me no great service by loving me despite all my extra pounds. I can't find any clothes that fit and, if I'm honest, I'm beginning to fear for my life."

His final sentence changed the course of my professional life: "Put me on whatever diet you want, deprive me of whatever food you want, anything, but not meat. I like meat too much."

I can still remember how I replied without the slightest hesitation: "Fine, since you like meat so much, come back tomorrow on an empty stomach and weigh yourself on my scales. Then, for the next 5 days, eat nothing but meat. However, avoid fatty meats like pork, lamb, and the fattier cuts of beef such as ribs or rib eye. Grill your meat and drink as much water as you can. Then come back in 5 days' time on an empty stomach and weigh yourself again."

"Okay, you have a deal."

Five days later, he was back. He had lost almost 12 pounds. I couldn't believe my eyes and neither could he. I felt somewhat concerned, but he looked great, more jovial than ever, saying he had rediscovered his well-being and had stopped snoring. He brushed aside my hesitations.

"I'll keep it up. I feel on top of the world. It works and it's a real treat."

And so he left for another 5 days of eating meat, promising me he would have blood and urine tests done.

When he came back, he had lost another 5 pounds, and, jubilant, he showed me his test results. His glucose, cholesterol, and uric acid levels were all perfectly normal.

In the meantime I had gone to the medical school library, where I spent time learning more about the nutritional properties of meat and other proteins.

When my patient returned 5 days later, still in tip-top shape and having shed another 4 pounds, I told him to add fish and seafood, which he accepted with good grace because he had explored all that meat had to offer.

When at the end of 20 days the scales registered a loss of 22 pounds, I ordered another blood test, which turned out to be just as reassuring as the first one. Playing my ace, I had him add the remaining categories of protein: dairy products, poultry, and eggs. However, to allay my concerns, I asked him to increase his water intake to 3 quarts—twelve 8-ounce glasses—a day.

He agreed to add vegetables, as I was beginning to worry that they had been absent from his diet for so long.

When he came back 5 days later, he had not lost an ounce. He used this as an argument to go back to his all-protein diet. I let him have his way on the condition that he alternate this regimen with 5-day periods that would include vegetables, arguing that otherwise he risked vitamin deficiency. He did not buy that argument, but he agreed because he was suffering from constipation due to the lack of fiber in his diet.

This is how the first phases of the Dukan Diet were born, as well as my interest in obesity and weight loss. My patient had changed the course of my studies and my professional life. I worked to improve the diet, creating an eating plan that seems to me today to be both the most appropriate for the particular psychological make-up of overweight people and also the most efficient for weight loss based on real food.

However, over the years, I have come to the bitter realization that even effective weight loss diets are not effective in the long term. At best, the dieter slowly and imperceptibly drifts off course; at worst the weight piles back on again, usually because of stress, setbacks, or other problems.

It was seeing how the vast majority of dieters inevitably lose this war against weight that led me to design a plan that protects the accomplishment of reaching the target weight. The job of this Consolidation phase is to reintroduce, in increments, the basic elements of proper eating and to control a body that, stripped of its reserves, would be bent on revenge. To allow enough time for this rebellious phase and to make the transition acceptable, I fixed a precise time limit for the second part of my plan, easy to calculate and in proportion to the weight lost: 5 days for every 1 pound lost.

However, once the Consolidation phase was over, I saw my patients' old habits gradually creep back, thanks to the pressures of metabolism and the inevitable resurgence of the need to compensate for life's miseries with those thick, creamy, sweet comfort foods that craftily overwhelm our defenses.

I therefore had to resort to a measure that is hard to even suggest to people, a rule that I dare to call "permanent," the kind of shackle that all overweight people—the obese or the just plain overweight—detest because it is there for good. However, this rule, which needs to be followed for the rest of one's life but which guarantees real weight stabilization, applies to *only a single day a week*—a day that is predetermined, whose structure cannot be changed or negotiated but which bears amazing results.

It was only then that I reached the Promised Land: genuine, long-lasting, unequivocal success built on four successive phases, each decreasing in intensity, which create a supportive and clearly signposted path that allows no escape. A short, strict Attack diet that gives lightning results is followed by a Cruise diet and sustained by a Consolidation phase, whose duration is proportionate to the weight lost. Finally, so that the weight you have achieved with such effort remains stable forever, there is a Stabilization phase, which includes a locking measure that is as specific as it is effective: *a single day a week devoted to dietary redemption*. This measure is designed to keep the rest of the week in balance, provided it stays by your side, like a loyal guard dog, for the rest of your life.

Finally, with these four successive diet phases, I achieved my first real lasting results. Now I no longer had only a fish to offer, but a whole course on how to fish, a comprehensive program that allows overweight people to be autonomous, lose weight quickly, and keep it off for good, and to do this all by themselves.

I have spent thirty-five years creating this beautiful tool for a limited number of people. Today I want a wider public to be able to access my program.

This program is for those of you who have tried everything, who have lost weight often—too often—and who are looking for a way not just to lose weight, but more important, to maintain those hard-earned results and live comfortably with the body you want and deserve.

So I dedicate this book and this method to all my patients, who have made my life as a doctor so fulfilling, and in particular to the very first of them, the overweight publisher.

THE BIRTH OF A FOUR-STEP DIET

The Dukan Diet

Thirty-five years have passed since my life-changing encounter with the obese gentleman. Since then, I have devoted my work to helping thousands of men and women lose pounds and stabilize their weight.

Like all my French medical colleagues, I was trained that calories counted and low-calorie diets were the way to lose weight. Every type of food was allowed in moderate quantities. Nowadays, what I know and practice I have learned through direct daily contact with flesh-and-blood human beings who have constant cravings to eat.

I very quickly realized that it was not by accident that an individual was overweight. Their appetite and their apparent lack of restraint were a camouflage concealing a need to find comfort in food. This need is all the more overwhelming as it is connected to our survival mechanisms, which are as archaic as they are instinctive. It soon became obvious to me that I could not make an overweight person lose weight and stay slim simply by giving sound advice, even if that advice was based on common sense and scientific research.

Support is what overweight people determined to lose weight really want and is what they need from a counselor or a method—support so that they are not left alone to face the ordeal of dieting, which deliberately goes against their own instinct for survival.

What overweight individuals are looking for is an outside will, a decision maker who walks ahead of them offering guidance and specific instructions, because what overweight people most hate and simply cannot do is decide for themselves when and how they are going to deprive themselves of food.

As for managing their weight, overweight individuals will admit without shame—and why should there be any?—that they are powerless when it comes to controlling what they eat. People from every social and economic background have all sat in front of me and described themselves as being astonishingly weak when it comes to food.

Obviously, most of them have found in food an easy "escape valve" through which they can release excess tension, stress, and life's all too frequent disappointments. Any logical, reasonable, and rational instructions just cannot stand up to those pressures—at least not for long.

During my years of practice, I have seen many diets come and go. From analyzing these diets and the reasons behind their various successes, as well as the efforts of my own patients, I am convinced of the following: Overweight people who want to lose weight need a fast-acting diet that brings immediate results, fast enough to strengthen and maintain their motivation. They also need precise goals, set by an outside instructor, with a series of levels to aim for so that they can see their efforts and compare them with the results expected. However, I have also observed the strength of my patients' resolve at certain times in their lives and then seen how easily they lose heart when the results do not match their efforts.

Most of the spectacular diets that rocketed to success in recent years did in fact have that fast-off-the-mark effect and delivered the promised results. Unfortunately, their instructions and guidance faded away once the book was closed, leaving the overweight individual once again all alone on the slippery slope of temptations, and the cycle would start all over again. Once the goal was reached, all these diets, even the most original and inventive, abandoned their followers with the same old commonsense advice about moderation and balance that a formerly overweight person will never manage to follow.

None of these famous diets managed to find a way of protecting and guiding individuals during the period that follows their weight loss, giving advice and precise, simple, and effective landmarks like those that made their initial program so successful.

People who have lost weight know instinctively that on their own, and without any support, they will not be able to preserve this victory. They also know that left to their own devices, the pounds will creep back on. They need instructions that are simple, specific, effective, and not too frustrating—guidelines that can be followed for the rest of their life.

Dissatisfied with the majority of the diets in vogue, which are only concerned with a dazzling but short-lived victory, and aware of the ineffectiveness of low-calorie diets and the kind of commonsense advice that despite all the evidence hopes to reform overeaters into careful eaters, I developed my own weight loss diet. Years of medical practice allow me to consider it both the most effective and easy-to-follow diet available today.

I realize that the preceding statement may make me appear immodest. But I will take that risk because it is my most heartfelt conviction, and not saying so in the face of the growing scourge of weight control problems would amount to a failure to assist people in danger.

The Dukan Diet takes into account everything that is essential for the success of any weight loss program:

- It offers overweight people trying to lose weight a system with specific instructions that get them on track, with stages and objectives, leaving no room for ambiguity or deviation.
- The initial weight loss is substantial and sufficiently rapid to launch the diet and instill lasting motivation.
- It is a low-frustration diet. Weighing food portions and calorie counting are banned, and it allows you total freedom to eat a certain number of popular foods.
- It is a comprehensive weight loss program, an integrated whole that you either take or leave.

The diet can be broken down into four successive phases:

1. *The Attack phase.* The initial Attack phase is a pure protein diet that creates a stunning kick start, almost as quick as fasting or powdered protein diets but without their drawbacks.

2. *The Cruise phase.* In the Cruise phase, pure protein days alternate with days in which you eat pure proteins plus certain allowed vegetables. This phase lets you reach your chosen weight.

3. *The Consolidation phase.* The Consolidation phase is designed to prevent the rebound effect that occurs after any rapid weight loss. This is a period of high vulnerability when the body has a tendency to very easily regain those lost pounds. The duration of this phase is based on a precise formula: 5 days for every pound lost.

4. *The Permanent Stabilization phase.* Permanent weight stabilization is based on three simple safety measures that are easy to follow but which are indispensable if the weight loss is to be maintained: The pure protein phase of the diet must be followed 1 set day per week—for example, every Thursday—for the rest of your life; do not use elevators or escalators; and take 3 tablespoons of oat bran a day. These three rules are non-negotiable, but they are sufficiently specific and effective for you to stick to them over a long period of time.

THE THEORY BEHIND THE DUKAN DIET

Before discussing the diet in detail and explaining exactly how it works and why it is so effective, I want first to give you an outline of the whole four-phase program to make clear from the outset precisely for whom the diet is intended, along with any possible contraindications.

One of the major merits of the Dukan Diet is its educational value. It allows you to learn in real life and with your own body the relative importance of each food group from the order in which they are integrated into the diet. That is, the diet starts with vital foods, then introduces, in succession, indispensable foods, essential foods, and important foods, finishing off with unnecessary but pleasurable foods.

The Dukan Diet provides a system of perfectly interwoven instructions that will clearly and directly set you on the right track, avoiding the need for that never-ending effort of willpower that can slowly undermine your determination.

I will be giving these instructions to you in four successive diet plans. The first two make up the actual weight loss stage, and the second two ensure that the weight loss you achieve is consolidated and then permanently stabilized.

1. The Attack Phase: The Pure Protein Diet

The Attack phase is the conquest phase. Here dieters are always extremely motivated. They are looking for a diet plan that, however arduous it might be, meets their expectations in terms of effectiveness and quick results and that allows them to tackle their weight problem head-on. The length of this phase depends on how much weight one wants to lose. The Attack phase can last as little as 1 day or as many as 10, with most people falling in the 2- to 7-day range.

The diet plan for this initial phase of the Dukan Diet, great for a fast-track approach, limits food to just one of the three food groups—namely, proteins.

Except for egg whites, no food is 100 percent protein. The pure protein diet of the Attack phase selects and groups together foods whose composition is as close as possible to pure protein, such as certain kinds of meat, fish, seafood, poultry, whole eggs, and nonfat dairy products.

Compared with low-calorie diets, the pure protein diet is a real war machine, a bulldozer that, if followed without fail, crushes all resistance. It is effective in the most difficult cases, in particular for premenopausal women suffering from water retention and bloating and for menopausal women. It is just as effective with dieters deemed to be resistant because they have tried and given up on too many diets or aggressive courses of treatment in the past.

2. The Cruise Phase: The Alternating Protein Diet

As its name indicates, this phase works by alternating two diets: the pure protein diet followed by the same diet to which any nonstarchy vegetable, raw or cooked, is added (see "100 Natural Foods That Keep You Slim," page 168). Each alternate cycle works like the injection-combustion cycle of a two-speed engine burning up its calorie quota.

In the alternating cycles of the Cruise phase you can eat the authorized "as much as you like" foods at any time of day and in the combination and quantity that best suits you. This gives you both complete freedom and an effective way of neutralizing your hunger by eating. Satisfaction through quantity makes up for any lack of variety.

Later I will discuss the precise timing for the alternating pattern of the Cruise phase, which will depend on how much weight you want to lose, how many diets you have already attempted, your age, and your level of motivation.

The Cruise phase must be followed *without* a break until your target weight is reached. Although influenced in part by previous bad experiences, the alternating protein diet is still one of the diets least affected by resistance induced by previous attempts at weight loss.

3. The Consolidation Phase: The Transition Diet—5 Days for Every Pound Lost

After you have achieved your goal weight comes the soothing phase of the Dukan Diet. Its purpose is to get you eating a wider variety of foods again, while avoiding the traditional rebound effect that occurs after losing a lot of weight. When you lose weight, your body tries to put up resistance. It reacts to its reserves being plundered by gradually reducing its energy output and, above all, by assimilating and getting as much energy as possible from any food that is eaten.

The successful dieter is therefore sitting on a volcano: Your body is just waiting for the right moment to win back its lost reserves. A large meal that before you reached this phase of the Dukan Diet would have had little effect will now, toward the end of the diet, have far-reaching consequences.

This is why the Consolidation phase opens up to include foods that are richer and more gratifying, but their variety and quantity will be limited so your body's metabolism can adjust to your new weight. Think of it as the first step in stabilizing your weight loss.

In the Consolidation phase, you will be adding 2 slices of bread and 1 portion of fruit and cheese into your daily diet, along with 2 servings of carbohydrates and 2 "celebration" meals a week.

The purpose of the Consolidation phase is to avoid the explosive rebound that is the most immediate and one of the most frequent reasons for failure in weight loss diets. It is now necessary to introduce foods as significant as bread, fruit, cheese, and some starches as well as certain unnecessary but extremely pleasurable dishes or foods. These added foods must, however, be introduced in a certain order to avoid the continual risk of slipping backward and to protect your weight loss. How long this phase lasts depends on how much weight has been lost—a very simple calculation based on 5 days for every pound lost.

4. The Permanent Stabilization Phase: Ultimate Long-Term Weight Control

Having lost weight and avoided any rebound by following the rules of the first three phases of the Dukan Diet, you may sense instinctively that your victory is fragile, and you may fear that, without support, sooner or later—more often sooner rather than later—you will be at the mercy of your old demons. One thing you may be even more certain of is that, when it comes to food, you may never acquire the discipline most nutritionists recommend as the way guaranteed to maintain weight loss. However, the Stabilization phase is designed to give you a way to maintain your hard-won goal: the original pure protein diet of the Attack phase—the most effective and the strictest weapon of my program—once a week, every Thursday, for the rest of your life.

As paradoxical as this might seem, once you have reached your desired weight, you are quite capable of making this effort 1 day a week because it is a very precise rule and because 1 day a week is a very limited amount of time. And, above all, this specific and non-negotiable rule bears immediate fruit, allowing you to eat normally for the other 6 days of the week without putting any weight back on.

THE DUKAN DIET SUMMARIZED

THE ATTACK PHASE: Pure Proteins
Length: 2 to 7 days, with the average being 5 days

THE CRUISE PHASE: 100 Unlimited Foods in Alternation
Average length: 3 days for each pound you want to lose

THE CONSOLIDATION PHASE:
Average length: 5 days per pound lost

THE PERMANENT STABILIZATION PHASE:
1 pure protein day every Thursday for life
No more elevators and escalators
3 tablespoons of oat bran a day

SOME USEFUL INFORMATION ABOUT NUTRITION

The CFP Trio:
Carbohydrates—Fats—Proteins

All food is made up of only three nutrients: carbohydrates, fats, and proteins. Every food gets its taste, texture, and nutritional interest from the particular way that these three elements combine.

Calories Are Unequal in Quality

Once upon a time, nutritional experts were only interested in the caloric value of foods and meals and based their weight loss diets entirely on calorie-counting, which explains why for so long diets failed without any apparent explanation.

Today, experts have abandoned this approach and instead are more interested in where the calories come from, the type of food providing the calories, the mix of nutrients that makes up the mass of chewed food, and even the time of day when the calories are taken in.

It can be proved that the body does not treat 100 calories provided by white sugar in the same way as it does 100 calories from oil or fish. Also the ultimate benefit of these calories after they are assimilated varies widely, depending on their origin.

The same holds true for the time of day these calories are consumed. It is now commonly agreed that the body burns up morning calories more efficiently than midday calories and even more efficiently than evening calories. Leaving aside the fact that it is specifically adapted to the overweight person's specific profile, the effectiveness of the Dukan Diet's four-phase plan can be explained by the very careful selection of nutrients that make up the foods I recommend, in particular the huge importance given to proteins during the Attack phase as well as during the Stabilization phase.

Carbohydrates

Carbohydrates have always supplied humans, whatever the place, era, or culture, with over 50 percent of our energy ration.

For thousands of years, apart from fruit and honey, the only carbohydrates we consumed were what we now call "slow sugars"—whole grains and starchy vegetables like root vegetables and legumes. What sets these "slow sugar" carbohydrates apart from refined carbohydrates—such as white rice, white bread, and foods containing refined sugar—is that they are absorbed gradually. "Slow sugar" carbohydrates raise the body's sugar levels only moderately, and thus do not cause reactive insulin surges and the resulting harmful repercussions on health—specifically, weight gain.

Since we discovered how to extract white sugar from sugar cane and then from sugar beets, human food has undergone profound changes, with an ever-increasing intake of sweet foods and refined carbohydrates. Providing excellent fuel, these types of carbohydrates are highly suitable for athletes, manual workers, and teenagers. But for the vast majority of sedentary people who make up most of today's societies they are far from useful.

High-carbohydrate foods that sabotage diets include

- White sugar and all its derivatives, such as candy and other sweets, are pure carbohydrates and absorbed in no time at all.
- Starchy foods, even if they do not taste sweet, are just as rich in carbohydrates. They include flour products (bread, in particular white bread, crackers, biscuits, cereals, and the like), pasta, potatoes, peas, legumes, lentils, and beans.
- The fruits containing the most carbohydrates are bananas, cherries, and grapes.
- Wine and all alcohol, including beer, spirits, or any food or drink containing alcohol.
- Pastries—are a delicious combination of flour and sugar, and, even worse, of fat.

Carbohydrates contain only 4 calories per gram but are usually eaten in such large quantity that the calories soon mount up. Carbohydrate calories are also totally assimilated, which increases their energy yield. Furthermore, we digest starch and flour products slowly, producing fermentation and gas, which causes bloating as unpleasant as it is unattractive.

Carbohydrates so energy-rich and easily available, and they have such a pleasant taste that they are often used as comfort foods. And, as for sweet foods, some people snack on them compulsively. Our affinity for sweet tastes is in part innate, but most psychologists agree that lengthy conditioning starting in childhood makes sweet flavors gratifying as they are associated with rewards.

Finally, carbohydrates are almost always the cheapest foods available, which is why they are served at everyone's table, from the richest to the poorest.

As far as the body's metabolism is concerned, carbohydrates help the secretion of insulin, which in turn encourages fat to be produced and stored.

For all these reasons, for a long time, people predisposed to being over-weight were instructed to be wary of carbohydrates. Nowadays, they are told instead to be wary of the fat content in foods, which—and rightly so—has now become the overweight person's most deadly enemy. However, this is not a reason to lower one's guard in respect to carbohydrates, especially during the Attack phase.

The Dukan Diet excludes carbohydrates completely during the Attack phase. In the Cruise phase and until the desired weight has been reached, it only allows vegetables with extremely low sugar levels (see "Vegetables You Can and Cannot Eat," page 68). Carbohydrates make a comeback during the Consolidation phase, but it is only during the final Stabilization phase, 6 days out of 7, that total restriction is lifted.

Fats

Fats are the absolute enemy of anyone trying to be slim, as they represent the most concentrated form in which surplus energy is stored. Eating fats means you are eating an animal's energy reserves, which, in theory as in practice, improve your chances of increasing your weight.

Since the Atkins Diet appeared, opening the way for eating immoderate amounts of fat by demonizing carbohydrates, many diets have adopted this point of view. However, this approach was quite clearly a major mistake for two reasons: (1) cholesterol and triglyceride levels rise dangerously; (2) mistrust of fats is gone, and once gone it makes any form of stabilization impossible.

There are two major sources of fats: animal and vegetable. Animal fat, found in a virtually pure state in lard, is very much present in pork products such as pâtés, salamis, sausages, hot dogs, and meat spreads. Lamb and mutton and certain poultry, such as goose and duck, have a plentiful supply. Beef is not as fatty, especially those cuts that can be grilled. Only ribs and the rib eye are really rich in fat. Butter, which comes from the creamy top of milk, is practically a pure fat. The fat content of heavy cream is around 36 percent.

The five fish with the most fat, easily recognizable by their rich taste and blue skin, are sardines, tuna, salmon, mackerel, and herring. But remember that these fish are no fattier than ordinary steak, and the fat of coldwater fish is rich in omega-3 fatty acids, a known safeguard against cardiovascular disease.

Vegetable fats are, for the most part, represented by the long list of plant and nut oils and fruits such as avocado. Oil is even fattier than butter. Although some oils like olive, canola, or sunflower oils have nutritional qualities that have been proved to protect the heart and arteries, they all have the same caloric value and should be banned from any weight loss diet, avoided during the Consolidation phase, and eaten sparingly during the final Stabilization phase. Peanuts, walnuts, hazelnuts, pistachios, and macadamia nuts are snacks that are often eaten with a cocktail; their combination with alcohol greatly increases the calorie intake of the meal to follow.

For those who want to be slim, and in particular for those who are trying to lose weight, fats represent every danger possible.

- Fats contain, by far, the most calories—9 calories per gram (more than double the calories in carbohydrates, which provide only 4 calories per gram).
- Fats are very rich foods and so are rarely eaten alone. Oil, butter, and heavy cream are often associated with bread, starch, pasta, or salad dressings; the combination increases the overall calorie count considerably.
- Fats are not assimilated as quickly as fast sugars, but they are assimilated far more quickly than proteins, and thus their comparative energy contribution increases accordingly.
- Fatty foods reduce our appetite only moderately, and snacking on them, rather than on proteins, does not reduce your desire for a large meal afterward or delay the time before you next feel hungry.
- Finally, animal fats with high amounts of fatty acids—butter, sausages, dried meats, and fatty cheeses—pose a potential threat to the heart. For this reason, they cannot be consumed without restriction, as has been the case with the Atkins Diet and other regimes inspired by it.

Proteins

Proteins are the third universal food group. The foods richest in proteins come from the animal kingdom. Their most abundant source is meat.

Among animal meat, beef is especially high in protein. The leaner cuts are extremely low in fat, but just as rich in protein. Mutton and lamb are visibly more marbled, and this fat reduces their protein content. Finally, some cuts of pork, which are even fattier, are not rich enough in protein to belong to the elite group of protein foods.

Organ meats like liver, kidneys, tongue, sweetbreads, chicken hearts, and tripe are very rich in protein and low in fat and carbohydrates. However, liver contains a small dose of sugar.

Poultry, with the exception of domestic goose and duck, is a relatively lean meat very rich in protein, especially turkey and chicken breast.

Fish, particularly lean white-fleshed fish like sole, skate, cod, sea bass, or tilapia are a gold mine of proteins with a very high nutritional value. Coldwater fish such as salmon, tuna, sardines, and mackerel have fattier flesh, which slightly reduces their protein content, but they nevertheless remain excellent sources of protein and greatly promote cardiovascular health.

Shellfish and other types of seafood are lean and carbohydrate-free, and rich in protein. Some, like shrimp and scallops, are often not allowed on weight loss diets because of their high cholesterol level, but that substance is concentrated in the "coral" (eggs or ovaries) of the animal's head and not its flesh, which means that you can eat shrimp, crab, and lobster without restriction as long as you take the precaution of removing the coral first.

Eggs are an interesting source of protein. The yolk contains fats and enough cholesterol that should you be predisposed to high cholesterol, you should avoid excessive consumption of the yolk. On the other hand, egg white is the purest and most complete known form of protein, which gives it the status of benchmark protein, as it is used to classify all other proteins.

Plant proteins are found in most cereals and legumes, but these are far too rich in carbohydrates to be included in a diet whose effectiveness depends on the purity of proteins. Furthermore, apart from soy, these plant proteins are desperately short of certain vital amino acids, so they cannot be used exclusively over a prolonged period of time.

So how can we be vegetarian? If it means not eating anything from an animal that has been raised and slaughtered for us to eat, but consuming eggs and dairy products, this is sufficient for people who are not trying to lose weight. If vegetarian means eating only vegetables, my diet becomes very hard to follow, as there is no other choice but to use incomplete vegetable proteins that have to be very cleverly teamed up with cereals and legumes to ensure that all amino acids are consumed, because without all amino acids, it is impossible for the body to produce vital proteins.

Man Is a Carnivorous Hunter

It is important to realize that humans emerged from their animal condition by becoming carnivorous. Our apelike ancestors, like today's great anthropoid apes, were essentially vegetarians, even if, occasionally, certain apes hunted other animals for food. Indeed, it was by becoming group hunters and meat eaters that humans were able to acquire uniquely human faculties. The human body possesses a whole system for digestion and elimination that still allows us today to eat unlimited quantities of meat and fish.

We are designed to eat meat, fish, and poultry, as far as both our metabolism and psychology are concerned. Yes, it is possible to live without hunting and without eating meat, but by doing so we give up a part of what our nature expects, and we lessen the emotional effect our body is programmed to produce when we give it what it expects. What I am saying to you here may seem trivial, but it is absolutely crucial, as the purpose of any living creature, whether animal or human, is to live in such a way that what it does fits with why it has been made that way.

Digestion, Calorie Loss, and Satisfaction

Of all the food categories, the digestion of proteins is the most time consuming. It takes over three hours to break down and assimilate proteins.

The reason for this is simple: protein molecules are long chains with well-soldered links, and to break down their resistance requires the combination of good chewing and the simultaneous attack of various gastric, pancreatic, and biliary juices.

This long process of calorie extraction taxes the system; it has been calculated that to obtain 100 calories from a protein food, the system must use 30 calories. We can say that the specific dynamic action of proteins is 30 percent, while it is only 12 percent for fats and just 7 percent for carbohydrates.

What we should remember from this is that when someone wanting to lose weight consumes meat, fish, or nonfat yogurt, the person has to work hard to simply digest and assimilate the food, and the calories they use doing this reduces the energy absorbed from the meal. This really works in the favor of anyone wanting to lose weight. We will explore this process at greater length when we explain how the pure protein diet works. What is more, this slow rate of digestion and assimilation delays the process of emptying the stomach and increases our sense of "feeling full" and our sense of satisfaction.

The Only Vital and Indispensable Nutrient at Every Meal

Of the three universal food groups, only proteins are indispensable for our existence. Carbohydrates are the least necessary nutrient, because our bodies can produce glucose—that is, sugar—from meat or fat. When we are deprived of food or are dieting, we draw upon our fat reserves, transforming them into the glucose that is vital for our muscles and brain. The same goes for fats: an overweight person is expert in both making and storing them.

On the other hand, we do not have the metabolic means to synthesize proteins. Just being alive and ensuring that our muscular system is maintained, that our red blood cells are renewed, that wounds heal, that hair grows, and even that memory functions—all these vital operations require proteins, a minimum of 1 gram per day for every 2 pounds of body weight.

Whenever there is not enough protein, the body is forced to draw upon its reserves, mainly the muscles, but it also uses skin or even bones. This is what happens when unreasonable diets are followed, such as juice fasts or the Beverly Hills Diet, which allows unlimited quantities of exotic fruits.

Recently, some diets have led people to believe that our bodies can be detoxified by eating just fruit and vegetables for a few days. When you realize it has been scientifically proved that after eight hours without good-quality proteins, the body has to draw upon its own muscle reserves to ensure its vital functions, you can understand just how inappropriate such ideas are.

Anyone wanting to lose weight should therefore realize that however restrictive the diet, it should never supply the body with less than 1 gram of protein per day for every 2 pounds of body weight, and, most important, protein intake should be evenly distributed over the day's three meals. A meager breakfast, lunch consisting of a pastry and a bar of chocolate, then pizza for dinner with fruit for dessert are all meals that lack protein and will make your skin dull and impair your body's general strength.

The Low-Calorie Value of Proteins

A gram of protein provides only 4 calories, the same as sugar but half of what fat provides.

Only 50 percent of all meat, fish, and other food proteins are assimilated; the rest is waste or useless tissue. This means that 4 ounces of turkey or steak provide only 200 calories. When you take into account that your body has to contribute 30 percent of this caloric value—that is, 60 calories—just to assimilate it, only 140 calories are left from this tasty and filling food, the equivalent of 1 tablespoon of the dressing you deem so harmless when you add it to your salad.

A high-protein diet has two drawbacks:

- *Protein is expensive.* The cost of protein is relatively high— meat, fish, and seafood can easily make a dent in a modest budget. Eggs, poultry, and offal, like chicken livers, are more affordable but are still expensive. Fortunately, nonfat dairy products make it possible to get excellent quality protein at a price that allows us to offset the high cost of protein meals.

- *Protein produces waste products that must be eliminated.* When protein is digested, waste products, such as uric acid, remain in the system and have to be eliminated. In theory, eating higher amounts of protein foods would increase the amount of waste products and cause discomfort to certain people. In fact, the human organs, and particularly the kidneys, have mechanisms for elimination and are perfectly suited to this task. But for the kidneys to work efficiently, it is absolutely necessary that they have an increased quantity of water. The kidneys will filter and remove uric acid from our blood, provided that we increase our normal consumption of water.

I had the opportunity to review sixty cases of patients suffering from either gout or uric acid kidney stones. They followed a protein-rich diet and also agreed to drink 3 quarts of water a day. Those who were already following treatment continued with it; the others, who were not on a treatment plan, did not add any medication. During the diet there was not a single case of uric acid levels rising; in fact a third of the patients saw their levels go down.

It is therefore essential when following a protein-rich diet to keep drinking water, especially during the protein-only phase. This is an opportune moment to deal with the accusations leveled against proteins by those who spread the idea that protein-rich foods can strain and even damage the kidneys. These same people have stated that even water can be toxic for the kidneys if you drink 1½ quarts per day. In thirty-five years of working with my diet and its unrestricted protein intake and insisting that my patients must drink at least 1½ quarts of water per day, I have never had a problem with a patient. I have even worked with thirty patients who, despite having only one kidney, lost weight without having any change in their renal markers. Apart from the usual prophets of doom, there are also jealous and troublemaking people—in particular, people who could do with losing weight themselves but lack the will to do so—who try to stop others from having a go. To such people I say, Come and join us, and let's drink a glass of water together!

Conclusion

Let's highlight some of the fundamental principles of a good weight loss diet:

- *Fats are the number one enemy.* Without doubt, fat both from animals and plants is the greatest enemy for anyone about to embark on a weight loss diet. Even before you start considering the fat content in meat or fish, just adding up the calories from the fat in cooking oil, sauces, marinades, dips, butter, and cream, as well as the fat found in cheese and sausages, is enough for fat to be awarded the prize for the highest source of calories. An effective, consistent diet therefore must start by reducing or eliminating fatty foods. You cannot lose your own fat by eating fat from other sources!
- *Animal fats pose a risk for the cardiovascular system.* You must also realize that animal fats alone contain cholesterol and triglycerides. Animal fats need to be reduced if there is any likelihood of cardiovascular risk or high cholesterol.
- *Simple carbohydrates are enemy number two.* For anyone wanting to lose weight, simple carbohydrates are their other enemy. I'm not speaking of the slow sugars found in whole grains or legumes, but of simple sugars like table sugar, which are assimilated quickly and trigger the pancreas to produce large amounts of insulin which in turn increases appetite and fat storage. Simple sugars are delicious to snack on, but their sweet taste can make you forget just how high their calorie concentration is.
- *Proteins have a moderate caloric value.* Proteins have only 4 calories per gram.

- *The calories in proteins cannot be completely assimilated.* Those foods richest in proteins, like meat or fish, are interwoven with connective tissue and are therefore very resistant to digestion, which means they are not completely assimilated. For overweight people, who by definition are great calorie assimilators, able to get the most out of anything they eat, this is manna from heaven, as it means they cannot extract all the calories in proteins.

- *It takes energy to digest and assimilate proteins.* If we subtract the energy needed for digesting proteins from the energy that protein foods contribute, 30 percent of their calories is saved, far more than with all other foods.

- *2 to 3 ounces of pure protein are needed daily.* Never go on a diet with fewer than 2 or 3 ounces of pure protein per day as it will rob you of muscle tissue and make your skin dull.

- *Drinking 1½ quarts of water a day eliminates protein's waste products.* Do not worry about uric acid, protein's natural waste product. You will eliminate it entirely by drinking 1½ quarts of water a day.

- *Proteins keep you from feeling hungry.* Remember that the more slowly a food is assimilated, the longer it takes for you to feel hungry again. Sweet foods are absorbed and assimilated the most rapidly, then fatty foods, and, after them, proteins. Those of you who constantly have food on your mind can draw your own conclusions.

PURE PROTEINS

The Driving Force Behind
the Dukan Diet

The Dukan Diet program is made up of four successive diets, designed so that they guide overweight people to their desired weight and keep them there. These four diets, which gradually include more foods, have been specially devised to accomplish the following, in chronological order:

- With the first diet, a lightning start and an intense and stimulating weight loss
- With the second diet, a steady, regular weight loss that takes you straight to your desired weight, your own True Weight
- With the third diet, consolidation of this newly achieved but still unstable weight, lasting for a fixed period of time—5 days for every pound lost
- With the fourth diet, permanent stabilization of your achieved weight, in return for three simple, concrete, guiding, extremely effective but non-negotiable measures to be followed for the rest of your life: protein Thursdays, no more elevators or escalators, and 3 tablespoons of oat bran a day

Each of the four diets has a specific effect and a particular mission to accomplish, but all four draw their force and their graduated impact from using pure proteins: pure proteins only during the Attack phase; proteins combined with vegetables during the Cruise phase; proteins in a more varied diet during the Consolidation phase, and, finally, 1 pure protein day a week again in the Stabilization phase.

The Attack phase gets its jump start by using the protein diet in its purest form for an average of 2 to 7 days, depending on the individual.

Alternating pure proteins with proteins and vegetables gives power and rhythm to the Cruise phase, which leads you straight to your desired weight.

The Consolidation phase is the period of transition between hard-line dieting and a return to normal eating.

And finally, in the Stabilization phase, the pure protein diet, followed for just 1 day a week for the rest of your life, guarantees permanent stabilization of your weight. In exchange for this occasional effort, for the other 6 days of the week you will be able to eat without guilt or any particular restriction.

How does the pure protein diet work? All will be explained in this chapter.

This Diet Provides Only Proteins

Where do you find pure proteins? Proteins form the fabric of living matter, both animal and vegetable, so they are found in most known foods. But to develop its unique action and full potential, the protein diet has to be composed of elements as close as possible to pure protein. In practice, other than egg whites, no food is this pure.

Whatever their protein content, vegetables are still too rich in carbohydrates. This includes all cereals, legumes, and starchy foods, and even soybeans. Though known for their protein quality, soybeans are too fatty and rich in carbohydrates.

Some animal proteins are also too high in fat. This is the case with pork, mutton and lamb, some poultry, such as duck and goose, and some cuts of beef and veal.

There are, however, a certain number of foods of animal origin that, without attaining the level of pure protein, come close to it and will be the main players in the Dukan Diet.

- Lean cuts of beef, no ribs, spare ribs, and cuts used for braising or stewing
- Lean cuts of veal
- Lean cuts of pork
- Game, such as venison, and some exotic meats, such as ostrich
- Poultry, except for domestic duck and goose
- All fish, including oily fish, whose fat helps protect the heart and arteries so they can be included here
- All other seafood
- Eggs, even though the small amount of fat in the yolk taints the purity of the egg white
- Nonfat dairy products. Though very rich in protein and totally fat-free, they may, nevertheless, contain a small amount of lactose, a natural milk sugar found in milk, just as fructose is found in fruit. They can, however, remain in the Dukan Diet's strike force because they have little lactose but lots of taste.

How Do Proteins Work?

The Purity of Proteins Reduces the Calories They Provide Every animal species feeds on foods made up of a mixture of the only three known food groups: proteins, carbohydrates, and fats. But for each species, there is a specific ideal proportion for these three food groups. For humans, the proportion is 5–3–2—that is, 5 parts carbohydrates, 3 parts fats, and 2 parts proteins, a composition close to that of mother's milk.

It is when our food intake matches this "golden proportion" that calories are most efficiently assimilated in the small intestine so that it is easy to put on weight.

On the other hand, all you have to do is change this proportion and the calories are not absorbed as well and the energy from the foods is reduced. Theoretically, the most radical modification conceivable, which would reduce most drastically the calories absorbed, would be to restrict our food intake to a single food group.

In practice, even though this approach has been tried out in the United States with carbohydrates (the Beverly Hills Diet allowed unlimited quantities of exotic fruits) or fats (the Eskimo diet), it is hard to eat only sugars or fats, and doing so has serious repercussions for our health. Too much sugar allows diabetes to develop easily, and too much fat, apart from our inevitable disgust, would pose a major risk to the cardiovascular system. Furthermore, proteins are essential for life and if the body does not get them it raids its own muscle for them.

If we are to eat from one single food group, the only possibility is lean proteins—a satisfactory solution as far as taste is concerned. It also avoids the risk of clogging up the arteries, and by definition it excludes protein deficiency.

When you manage to introduce a diet limited to protein foods, the body cannot use all the calories contained in the food. The body takes the proteins needed for survival and for the vital maintenance of its organs (muscles, blood cells, skin, hair, nails), and it makes poor and scant use of the other calories provided.

Assimilating Proteins Burns Up a Lot of Calories To understand the second property of proteins that makes the Dukan Diet so effective, you need to familiarize yourself with the idea of the specific dynamic action (SDA) of foods. The SDA of a food represents the effort or energy that the body has to use to break down the food until it is reduced to its basic unit, which is the only form in which it can enter the bloodstream. How much work this involves depends on the food's consistency and its molecular structure.

When you eat 100 calories of white sugar, the work the body must do to absorb it burns up only 7 calories, so 93 usable calories remain. Thus the SDA for carbohydrates is 7 percent.

When you eat 100 calories of butter or oil, assimilating them is a bit more laborious. The body burns 12 calories in absorbing them, leaving only 88 usable calories. Thus the SDA of fats is 12 percent.

Finally, to assimilate 100 calories of pure protein—egg whites, lean fish, or nonfat cottage cheese—the task is enormous. This is because protein is composed of an aggregate of very long chains of molecules whose basic links, amino acids, are connected to each other by a strong bond that requires a lot more work to be broken down. It takes 30 calories just to assimilate the proteins, leaving only 70 usable calories. Thus the SDA of proteins is 30 percent.

Assimilating proteins makes the body work hard and is responsible for producing heat and raising our body temperature, which is why swimming in cold water after eating a protein-rich meal is inadvisable, for the change in internal body temperature can result in immersion hypothermia.

This characteristic of proteins, annoying for anyone desperate for a swim, is a blessing for overweight people who are usually so good at absorbing calories. It means they can save calories painlessly and eat more comfortably without any immediate penalty.

At the end of the day, after eating 1,500 calories worth of proteins, a substantial intake, only 1,050 calories remain after digestion. This is one of the Dukan Diet's keys and one of the reasons why it is so effective. But that's not all.

Pure Proteins Reduce Your Appetite Eating sweet foods or fats does create a superficial feeling of satiety, all too soon swept away by the return of hunger. Recent studies have proved that snacking on sweet or fatty foods does not delay your urge to eat again or reduce the quantities eaten at the next meal. On the other hand, snacking on proteins does delay your urge for your next meal and does reduce the amount that you then eat. What is more, eating only protein foods produces ketones, powerful natural appetite suppressants that are responsible for a lasting feeling of satiety. After 2 or 3 days on a pure protein diet, hunger disappears completely, and you can follow the Dukan Diet without the natural threat that weighs down most other diets: hunger.

Pure Proteins Fight Edema and Water Retention Certain diets or foods are known as being "hydrophilic"—that is, they encourage water retention and the bloating this causes. This is the case for mostly vegetable diets, rich in fruits, vegetables, and mineral salts. Protein-rich diets are the exact opposite. They are known to promote elimination through urine and, as such, provide a welcome purge or "drying out" for tissues gorged with water, which is a particular problem during the premenstrual cycle or during perimenopause.

The Attack diet, made up exclusively of pure proteins, best gets rid of water. This is particularly advantageous for women. When a man gains weight, it is mostly because he overeats and stores his surplus calories in the form of fat. For a woman, how she puts on weight is often more complex and bound up with water retention, which prevents diets from working properly.

At a certain time during the menstrual cycle—in the four or five days before a period starts—or at certain key times in a woman's life—such as puberty, perimenopause, or even in the prime of her sexual life if she has hormonal disorders—a woman, and especially one who is overweight, begins to retain water and starts to feel spongy, bloated, and puffy faced in the morning. She is unable to remove rings from her swollen fingers, her legs feel heavy, and her ankles swell. This weight gain is reversible, but it can become chronic.

Even women who diet in order to avoid this bloating are surprised to find that during these periods of hormonal surge, all the little things that worked before no longer have any effect. In all these cases, a diet of pure proteins such as those found in my program's Attack phase have a decisive and immediate effect. In a few days, sometimes even in a matter of hours, water-soaked tissues begin to dry up, leaving a feeling of well-being and lightness that shows up immediately on the scales and greatly boosts motivation.

Pure Proteins Boost Your System's Resistance Before tuberculosis was eradicated through antibiotics, one of the traditional treatments was to overfeed patients by significantly increasing the amount of proteins in their diet. At the beginning of the twentieth century, at Berck in northern France, one of the top centers for treating tuberculosis, teenagers were even forced to drink animal blood. Today, sports coaches and trainers advocate a protein-rich diet for athletes who demand a lot from their bodies. Doctors give the same advice to increase resistance to infection, for anemia, or to speed up the healing of wounds.

It is advisable to make use of this advantage, because any weight loss, no matter how small, will weaken the body. I have personally seen that the Dukan Diet's Attack phase is the most stimulating phase. Some patients have even told me that it had a euphoric effect, both mentally and physically, and that this happened from the end of the second day.

Pure Proteins Enable You to Lose Weight Without Losing Muscle or Skin Tone There is nothing surprising in this observation when you realize that the skin's elastic tissue, as well as muscle, is made up essentially of proteins. A diet lacking in proteins forces the body to use its own muscles and the skin's proteins, so the skin loses its elasticity. Combined, these effects cause aging of the skin, the hair, and even one's general appearance, which friends and family soon notice, and which can be enough to make you stop the diet early.

Conversely, a protein-rich diet and, even more so, a diet made up exclusively of proteins like the Dukan Diet's Attack phase, has no reason to attack the body's reserves because the body is being given massive protein supplies. Under these conditions, the weight loss is rapid, muscle firmness is maintained, and the skin glows, allowing you to lose weight without looking older.

This particular feature of the Dukan Diet might seem of secondary significance to young women with firm muscles and wrinkle-free skin, but it is very important for those women approaching their fifties and therefore menopause, or those who have less muscle structure or fine and delicate skin. This is especially important because, and it has to be said here, there are too many women nowadays who manage their figures guided solely by their scales. Weight cannot and should not be the sole issue. Radiant skin, healthy-looking hair, muscle strength, and general body tone are criteria that contribute just as much to a woman's appearance.

This Diet Must Include a Lot of Water

The Importance of Drinking Water

Opinions and rumors circulate about how much water you should drink, but almost always there is some kind of "authority" telling you today the exact opposite of what you heard yesterday. However, this water issue is not simply a marketing concept for diets; it is a question of great importance.

To simplify things, it may seem essential to burn calories so that our fat reserves melt away; but this combustion, as necessary as it is, is not enough. Losing weight is as much about eliminating waste as it is about burning fat.

Would you do a load of laundry or wash the dishes without rinsing them? It is the same with losing weight. A diet that does not involve drinking a sufficient quantity of water is a bad diet. Not only is it ineffective, it leads to the accumulation of harmful waste.

Water Purifies the Body and Improves the Diet's Results Simple observation shows us that the more water you drink, the more you urinate and the greater the opportunity for the kidneys to eliminate waste derived from the food burned. Water is, therefore, the best natural diuretic. It is surprising how few people drink enough water.

The many demands in our busy day conspire to delay, then finally eliminate, our natural feeling of thirst, which no longer plays its part in warning us about tissue dehydration. Many women, whose bladders are smaller and more sensitive than men's, do not drink to avoid having to go to the bathroom constantly, or because it is awkward at work or on public transport, or because they do not like public restrooms.

However, what you may get away with under ordinary circumstances must change when you are following a weight loss diet.

Trying to lose weight without drinking water is not only toxic for the body, it can reduce and even completely block the weight loss so that all your work is for nothing.

Why?

Because the human engine that burns its fat while dieting functions like any combustion engine. Burned fuel (proteins) gives off heat and waste. If these waste products are not regularly eliminated by the kidneys, they will accumulate and, sooner or later, interrupt combustion and prevent any weight loss, even if you are following the diet scrupulously.

It is the same for a car engine with a clogged exhaust pipe, or a fire in a fireplace full of ashes. Both end up choking and dying from the buildup of waste. Sooner or later, bad nutrition and the accumulated effects of bad healthcare and extreme or unbalanced diets will make the overweight person's kidneys become lazy. More than anyone else, overweight people need large quantities of water to get their kidneys working efficiently again.

At the outset, drinking a lot of water may seem tedious and unpleasant, especially in wintertime. But if you keep it up, the habit will grow on you. Then, encouraged by the pleasant feeling of cleaning out your insides and, even better, of losing weight, drinking often ends up once again becoming something you want to do.

When They Are Combined, Water and Pure Proteins Act Powerfully on Cellulite This issue concerns women, as cellulite is a type of fat that, under hormonal influence, accumulates and remains trapped in the thighs, hips, and knees. Diets are very often powerless against it. I have discovered that the pure protein diet, together with a reduction in salt intake and an increase in consumption of mineral water (see "Which Water Should You Drink?," page 33) with a low mineral salt content, leads to a weight loss with moderate but genuine weight loss in the difficult areas, such as the thighs or the insides of the knees, and achieves the best overall reduction around the hips and thighs.

These results can be explained by the diuretic effect of proteins and the intense filtering undertaken by the kidneys made possible by the increased water intake. Water penetrates all tissues, even cellulite. It goes in, pure and clean, and comes out salty and full of waste. Adding the powerful effect of burning up pure proteins to this expulsion of salt and waste brings about definite, even if modest, results. This is a rare achievement and sets this diet apart from most others, which have no specific effect on cellulite.

When Should You Drink Water? People still cling to old wives' tales that would have you believe that it is best not to drink at mealtimes to avoid food's trapping the water. Not only does this idea have no physiological basis, in many cases it makes things worse. Not drinking while you eat, at a time when you naturally get thirsty and when drinking is so easy and enjoyable, may result in your suppressing your thirst. Then, when you are busy later on with your daily activities, you may forget to drink water for the rest of the day. During the Dukan Diet and especially during the alternating proteins phase, except in cases of exceptional water retention caused by hormonal or kidney problems, it is absolutely essential to drink 1½ quarts of water a day. If possible, drink mineral water, or take it in any other liquid form such as tea, herbal tea, or coffee.

Have a cup of tea at breakfast, a large glass of water midmorning, 2 more glasses and a coffee at lunch, 1 glass during the afternoon, and 2 glasses with dinner and you have easily downed 2 quarts. Many patients have told me that in order to drink when they were not thirsty, they got into the habit of drinking directly from the bottle, and this worked better for them.

Which Water Should You Drink? *Mineral water.* The most suitable waters for the pure protein Attack phase are mineral waters low in sodium, which are slightly diuretic and laxative. Among the best-known mineral waters are Evian, Poland Spring, Fiji Water, Voss, Saratoga Springs, and Perrier, the famous sparkling variety. You should avoid San Pellegrino, which is good but contains too much sodium to be drunk in large quantities.

Tap water. If you drink tap water, then continue to do so. It is far more important to drink enough water to get your kidneys working again than it is to worry about what is in the water you are drinking.

Tea. The same holds true for all the various sorts of teas, green teas, and herbal teas, especially in colder weather.

Diet soda. In the case of diet sodas, I consider them all to be great allies in the fight against weight problems (or excess weight) as long as they have no more than 1 calorie per glass. As far as I am concerned, not only do I allow them, but I recommend them and for several reasons.

First of all, diet sodas are often the best way to make sure you drink the 1½ quarts of liquid already mentioned. In addition, they have virtually no calories or sugar. Finally, and above all, a carbonated beverage like Diet Coke or Coca-Cola Zero, the market-leading brand, provides a clever mix of intense flavors, which can reduce the craving for sugar if used repeatedly by those who like snacking on sweet things.

Many of my patients have confirmed that diet sodas were fun and comforting when used as a part of their diet and actually helped them. The sole exception regarding diet sodas is in the case of a dieting child or teenager. It has been proved that substituting "fake" sugar barely reduces their craving for sugar. Furthermore, unlimited use of sweet-tasting carbonated drinks might form a habit of drinking without thirst and just for pleasure.

Water Is Naturally Filling As you know, we often associate the sensation of an empty stomach with being hungry, which is not entirely wrong. Water drunk during a meal and mixed with food increases the total volume of the food mass and stretches the stomach, creating the feeling of a full stomach, the first sign of satisfaction and satiety. This is another reason for drinking at mealtimes. However, experience proves that keeping the mouth busy works just as well in between meals—for example, during the danger zone in your day, between 5 p.m. and 8 p.m. A big glass of any liquid will often be enough to calm your hunger pangs.

Nowadays, the world's richest populations are confronting a new type of hunger: a self-imposed denial while surrounded by an infinite variety of foods that they dare not touch because of the risk to their health or because they have weight problems.

It is surprising to see that at a time when individuals, institutions, and pharmaceutical laboratories dream of discovering the perfect and most effective appetite suppressant, there are so many people for whom this is an issue. They still do not know about or even worse refuse to use a method as simple, pure, and inexpensive as drinking water to tame their appetite.

The Diet Has to Be Low in Salt

Kicking the Salt Habit

Salt is an element vital to life and present to varying degrees in every food, so adding salt at the table is always superfluous. Salt is just a condiment that improves the flavor of food, sharpens the appetite, and is all too often used purely out of habit.

A Low-Salt Diet Is Never Dangerous You could and even should live your whole life on a low-salt diet. People with heart and kidney problems or high blood pressure live permanently on low-salt diets without suffering harmful effects. However, people with natural low blood pressure and those who are used to using salt on their food should exercise caution.

A diet too low in salt, especially when combined with a large intake of water, can lower blood pressure. If your blood pressure is already naturally low, this can produce fatigue and dizziness if you get up quickly. People with low pressure should not go overboard with salt reduction and should limit their water intake to 1½ quarts per day.

On the Other Hand, Too Much Salt Leads to Water Retention In hot climates, salt pills are regularly distributed to workers so that they avoid dehydration.

However, many women, especially women intensely influenced by hormones during premenstrual or perimenopausal periods, or even during pregnancy, retain impressive amounts of water.

For these women, this water reduction diet par excellence works most effectively when as little salt as possible is absorbed, allowing the water to pass more quickly through the body

By the way, we often hear people complaining that they have put on 2 or even 4 pounds in one evening after a lapse in their diet. Sometimes a weight gain like this is not due to a real lapse. When we analyze exactly what was eaten, we can never track down the 18,000 calories of food required to produce these 4 extra pounds. It was simply the combination of an oversalty meal accompanied by wine, beer, or cocktails. Salt and alcohol combine to slow down the elimination of the water drunk. Never forget that 1 quart of water weighs about 2 pounds, and 2 teaspoons of salt are enough to retain this water in your body's tissues for a day or two.

This being the case, if during your diet you cannot avoid a professional dinner engagement or a family celebration that will force you to put aside the rules of the Dukan Diet, then at least avoid eating salty foods and drinking too much alcohol. And do not weigh yourself the next morning, because a sudden increase in weight may discourage you and undermine your determination and confidence. Wait until the following day—or, even better, 2 days—while returning to the diet, drinking mineral water with a low mineral content, and cutting back on salt. These three simple measures should be enough to get you back on track.

Salt Increases Appetite—Decreasing Your Salt Intake Decreases Your Appetite This is a simple observation. Salty foods increase salivation and gastric acidity, which in turn increase your appetite. Conversely, lightly salted foods have only a slight effect on digestive secretions and no effect on appetite. Unfortunately, the absence of salt reduces thirst, and thus when you follow the Dukan Diet, you need to accept that during the first days you will have to make yourself drink a large amount of liquid so that you boost your need for water and reestablish your natural thirst.

Forget Calories, Think Categories

The pure protein diet, the initial and principal driving force behind the four integrated diets that make up my program, is not like other diets. It is the only one to use just a single food group and one well-established category of foods with the highest protein content.

During the pure protein diet and throughout the whole program, any mention of calories and of calorie counting is to be avoided. Whether a few or many calories are eaten has little effect on the results; what counts is eating only the prescribed foods. So the actual secret of the program's first two weight loss phases is to eat a lot, even to eat in anticipation, before the hunger pangs take over. Hunger that turns into an uncontrollable craving that can no longer be appeased by pure proteins leads the careless dieter toward comfort foods with little nutritional value—sugary, creamy, rich, and destabilizing foods that nevertheless have a strong emotional power.

By following the Dukan Diet, you have replaced a calories system with a categories system. There is absolutely no need for you to count calories; all you need do is stay within the categories. But if you stray away from the list of permitted foods, you are no longer allowed to eat any quantity you like, and you will have to start counting how many calories you eat.

So this is a diet you cannot follow in half measures. It relies on the all-or-nothing law, which explains not only its metabolic effectiveness, but also its amazing impact on the psychology of an overweight person.

With a temperament that goes from one extreme to another, just as determined when making an effort and as easygoing when giving up, overweight people find in each of the four stages of my program an approach to suit them perfectly.

These affinities between the individual's psychological profile and the diet's structure create a synergy that is decisive for the dieter.

THE
DUKAN DIET
IN
PRACTICE

You have now reached the decisive moment of putting my program into practice. You now know everything you need to understand about how it works and the effectiveness of the four diets that make it up. In the introduction to the theory, I also tried to help you understand that people do not become overweight by accident. The pounds you have gained that you now want to get rid of are a part of you that you may want to deny, but they are nevertheless a part that is a reflection of your nature, of your psychology, and therefore of your identity.

The extra pounds you carry have as much to do with your personality, emotions, and feelings and your own particular way of using the pleasure from food to deal with life's small and large problems as they do with your genes, a family predisposition to put on weight, or the way your metabolism works.

That is to say, the problem is not as simple as it seems, and it explains why so many others, and maybe you too in the past, have failed. To struggle against a force as powerful and ancient as the need to eat obviously cannot be based simply on rationally learning about nutrition, or on the hope that you will achieve self-control on your own.

To stand any chance against the force of instinct, you have to fight it on its own ground, with means, language, and a strategy that come from the same instinctive level. Our need to feel desirable, our need for well-being, our fear of illness, our need to belong to a group, and our need to conform to prevailing style trends come from this level. Nowadays they are the only instinctive defense forces capable of motivating people to lose weight. But with the first signs of improvement, these motivations fade away. As soon as our self-image improves, our clothes no longer feel too tight, or we are able once again to climb stairs without losing our breath, these defenses are gone.

But above all, in order for a diet—or better, a comprehensive dieting program—to stand any chance of being adopted and followed by an overweight person, we need to use another area of instinct: the command of authority.

The recommendations for a weight loss program must therefore be formulated by an outside authority figure— another will that takes the place of an overweight person's will and that speaks with precise, non-negotiable instructions that are not open to interpretation and that, above all, are kept in a sustainable form for as long as the dieter intends to maintain the results.

The Dukan Diet is based on the remarkable effectiveness of consuming pure proteins, and it includes a whole system of foolproof instructions to channel and make the most of the psychology of the overweight person. In designing this diet, I also realized that a one-step plan was not adequate for such a complex task. I therefore devised a program with four successive diet phases, one following the other, a complete and coherent system that never, ever leaves the overweight person to face temptation and failure alone.

Recently I have realized that losing weight without incorporating exercise—the simplest and most natural exercise imaginable, so it becomes a part of your long-term routine—runs the risk of undermining this undertaking. I now no longer just recommend exercise, specifically walking, I *prescribe* it as I would medication. I will be discussing these exercise prescriptions in greater detail in a later chapter.

THE
ATTACK
PHASE

The Pure Protein Diet

However much weight is to be lost over whatever length of time, my program always starts with the pure protein diet, which creates a psychological trigger and a first decisive weight loss.

I will now review in detail all the foods you will use in this first phase, adding some advice to the description to make your personal choice easier.

How long does this initial Attack phase have to last? There is no standard reply for this extremely important question; how long it lasts depends on each individual. It primarily depends on how much weight you want to lose, but also on your age, how many previous diets you have tried, how motivated you are, and how you feel about proteins.

I will also give you very precise information about the results you can expect from the Attack diet, which obviously rely on the diet's being followed to the letter and for the correct length of time.

Finally, I will outline the various reactions you might encounter during this initial period.

- Pork: Lean cuts are permitted, such as tenderloin, loin roast, or well-trimmed center-cut chops.
- Lamb is not allowed in the Attack phase.

You can prepare all these meats as you like but without using any butter, oil, or cream, not even low-fat versions. However, if using a nonstick pan, you can rub the surface with a few drops of oil on a piece of paper towel to keep the flavor of the cooked meat without additional fat.

I recommend that you grill your meat, but these meats can also be roasted in the oven, cooked on a rotisserie, or even boiled. How well done or not you like your meat is up to you. But do remember that the longer the meat is cooked, the less fat there is, which comes closest to the Dukan Diet's ideal of pure protein.

You can also use lean ground meat prepared as burgers or as meatballs mixed with an egg, spices, capers, or pickles, and grilled or cooked in the oven. Raw meat is allowed (if you are completely confident of the source), tartare or carpaccio style, but it must be prepared without oil. Frozen beef burgers are allowed, but make sure that the fat content does not exceed 10 percent—15 percent is too rich for the Attack phase. You would do better to grind some lean meat yourself in your food processor, or cook the burger until most of the fat runs off.

I will remind you again that you can eat as much as you want.

Category 2: Organ Meats

Only liver (beef, veal, or poultry), kidneys, and tongue are allowed. Liver is rich in vitamins, which is very useful during a diet. Unfortunately, liver is also high in cholesterol, so it should be avoided if you have any cardiovascular problems.

Category 3: Fish

There is no restriction or limitation with this family of foods. All fish are allowed: lean or fat; white or oily; fresh, frozen, dried, or smoked; or canned (but not in oil or sauce containing fat).

Which Foods Are Allow

During the Attack phase, which can last from 2
lowed to eat foods from the eleven categories on t

From these categories, you can eat as much as y
suits you, with no limit and at whatever time of da
may also freely combine foods from any of these c

You can just select the foods you like, leaving t
extreme cases, you can eat from a single category
for 1 day.

The essential thing is to stick to this precisely def
that I have been prescribing it to people for many y
not left anything out. You must also realize that succ
foods, as small as the lapse may be, will be like punctu
a needle.

An apparently harmless lapse will be enough for
benefits of this precious freedom of being able to ea
just a tiny gain in variety, you will be forced for the
count your calories and restrict what you eat.

In short, the rule is simple and non-negotiable: Yo
erything on the following list, with complete freedo
is not on the list is forbidden, so forget about it for n
in the near future you will again be eating all the food
removed.

Category 1: Lean Meats

By lean meat, I mean beef, veal, lean pork, and game.

- Beef: All roasts or grilled beef are allowed—name
  tenderloin, sirloin, and roast beef; you must careft
  all types of ribs as they are too fatty.
- Veal: Recommended are veal cutlets and roast veal; v
  are allowed as long as you trim all the fat.
- Buffalo and venison are permitted.

- All fatty fish and oily fish are allowed, such as sardines, mackerel, bluefish, tuna, and salmon.
- All white and lean fish are also allowed, such as sole, halibut, cod, sea bass, mahi-mahi, tilapia, orange roughy, catfish, perch, skate, trout, flounder, and monkfish, as well as many other lesser-known varieties.
- Smoked fish is permitted, too. Smoked salmon, although greasy looking, is less fatty than a 90 percent fat-free steak. The same goes for smoked trout, tuna, eel, and haddock.
- Canned fish, very handy for quick meals or picnics, is allowed if it is in brine or water, such as tuna, salmon, mackerel, or sardines. Canned sardines in tomato sauce are also permitted.
- Finally, you are allowed to have surimi. Originally from Japan, these imitation crab sticks are made with very lean white-fleshed fish that has been pulverized and flavored with crab sauce and a little sugar. Many of my readers have an unfavorable opinion of this product. It is true that it is a processed food, but having researched into how it is produced, I have seen that it is of high nutritional quality, prepared from small white-fleshed fish on factory ships on the open sea. Others have pointed out to me that the labels mention carbohydrates. This is true but does not rule the product out, as the carbohydrates are starch that can be tolerated because of surimi's other qualities. The fat content is in fact very low.

Always cook your fish without oil or butter, but moisten it with lemon juice or a little soy sauce, and sprinkle with herbs and spices. Enjoy it baked, poached, or steamed.

Category 4: Shellfish

Here I include crustaceans and all shellfish: shrimp, crayfish, crab, lobster, scallops, oysters, clams, and mussels, as well as squid and octopus.

Keep these in mind and use them to add a festive touch to your menu and make it interesting and varied. They are also very filling and satisfying.

Category 5: Poultry

- All poultry is allowed except birds with flat bills, such as farm-reared goose and duck, provided you do not eat the skin. You can leave the skin on when cooking and remove it on your plate at the last moment so that the meat does not dry out.
- Chicken is the most popular poultry product and the most practical one for the pure protein Attack diet. Everything is allowed except the outside part of the wings, which is too fatty and cannot be separated from the skin. However, you should be aware that different parts of the chicken have different amounts of fat. The leanest part is the white breast meat, followed by the thigh, then the wing. Finally, the chicken should be as young as possible.
- Turkey in all forms is allowed, as are Cornish hens and quail. If you have access to game birds such as pheasant and wild duck, which is lean, these are also permitted.

Category 6: Low-Fat Ham, with Any Rind Cut Off, Smoked Turkey and Chicken, Dried Beef

For some time now, low-fat ham and smoked turkey or chicken has been available in supermarkets. They have a fat content between 2 and 4 percent. This is far below the fat content of lean meats and the leanest of fish. They are highly recommended and are very easy to use. They are perfect to take with you for lunch.

The same goes for thinly sliced dried beef and the Italian version, *bresaola,* which comes from dried beef fillet. These are very lean and tasty delicatessen products that unfortunately are also relatively expensive. Remember that deli hams and cured hams are not allowed, nor is smoked ham, which is even fattier.

Category 7: Eggs

Eggs can be eaten hard-boiled, soft-boiled, poached, or in an omelet, but always without any butter or oil. Unless you are sure of the source of your eggs, they should be cooked through; undercooked eggs carry the risk of salmonella. If you have access to pasteurized eggs, this will not be an issue. Egg substitutes, fresh, frozen, or powdered, can be an alternative to eggs if you want to cut your intake of fat and cholesterol, which are concentrated in the egg's yolk. These products, like Eggbeaters, or Better'n Eggs, contain 99 percent egg whites. The other one percent consists of undefined "natural flavor," coloring, spices, salt, onion powder, xanthan gum and guar gum.

To make your eggs more sophisticated and less monotonous, you can add shrimp or even some shredded crab. Try omelets with chopped onion or a few asparagus tips just for the flavor, ham, and spices. In a diet in which quantities are not restricted, eggs can be problematic because the yolks are high in cholesterol. Anyone with a high cholesterol level should consume no more than 3 or 4 egg yolks a week. But egg whites, a pure protein par excellence, can be eaten without restriction. You can make omelets using just one yolk for every two whites. Some people are allergic to eggs; of course they should avoid them.

If you are not allergic to eggs, do not have a high cholesterol count, and cook them without oil or butter, you may eat 2 eggs every day without running any risk during the brief Attack phase.

Category 8: Vegetable Proteins

In the last decade, I have noticed a reduction in the appetite for meat, especially among women. Vegetable proteins come from soy and wheat (gluten); most come from Asia, in particular Japan.

Here I will discuss seven foods that are very high in protein and low in fat. However, *note that only the first two—tofu and seitan—have the relationship between proteins, fats, and carbohydrates that allows them to be used in unlimited quantities*, like the foods in the seven previous categories. The last five—tempeh, soy steaks or vegetable burgers, textured soy protein (TSP), soy milk, and soy yogurt—are foods that I would reserve only for vegetarian readers who do not consume meat or fish. For nonvegetarians, these five foods should be thought of only as "tolerated foods," and used occasionally, assuming you are meeting your weight loss goals. See page 262 for more information about these "tolerated foods."

Tofu Tofu comes in several forms, the most common of which are silken and firm or extra firm, and is widely available in supermarkets as well as natural and health food stores.

> *Silken tofu* has the consistency of flan or yogurt. It can be found either with the refrigerated vegetables or in the dairy case. It is useful in making dessert and pastry recipes and quiches based on oat bran galettes (see recipe, page 54). It is also an interesting alternative in the preparation of sauces to replace mayonnaise, yogurt, or sour cream. Its consistency means that it can be whipped to act as a cream substitute.
>
> *Firm (or extra firm) tofu* has the consistency of semisoft cheese. It can be used in various forms: crumbled, grated, in small chunks, or as a purée for all kinds of main dishes, starters, and desserts. It is naturally tasteless but soaks up all the flavors of the foods surrounding it. It combines very well with chives, soy sauce, and mild spices. Use it in chunks in mixed salads or pureed in vegetable tarts made with oat bran.

Tofu benefits enormously from being marinated in the sauce of your choice for a few hours before cooking. To allow it to better soak up the flavor of the marinade, be sure to remove all its water by pressing it between two plates using a weight.

Firm tofu is stored like mozzarella, refrigerated in water that should be changed every 2 days, for not more than 10 days.

Tofu holds a favored position in the Dukan Diet. You can now find herbed tofu, curried tofu, and smoked tofu. You can find tofu dumplings, vegetarian sausages, stir fries, and ravioli made using tofu, all of very high quality and great flavor. A word of warning! Not all these dishes and presentations have been cooked in accordance with our dieting requirements, and you should look closely at their labeling in order to avoid those with a fat content of over 8 percent, and, of course, dishes like ravioli or dumplings are not suitable for the Attack phase of the diet.

Seitan Seitan, or "vegetable meat," is made with wheat protein rather than soy protein. Its resistant texture is reminiscent of meat, which allows it to be used in stews, prepared on skewers, or braised.

Seitan can be found ready to use, natural or flavored, in Asian stores, natural and health food stores, and some well-stocked supermarkets. While used primarily by vegetarians and vegans as a source of protein, I think it is high time for it to be introduced to a wider audience, especially people who are trying to lose weight.

On a nutritional level, seitan is a food extremely rich in protein (25 percent and low in calories (110 calories per 100 grams). It also contains very few carbohydrates, almost no fat, and no cholesterol. Use seitan by the date on the package; it can also be frozen for longer storage.

To cook seitan, pan-frying it gently in a covered nonstick pan over low heat will make it become more tender. Quick-frying it will make it hard. To maintain the best consistency and flavor, avoid using slices that are too thick. Think about marinating the slices in a mix of soy sauce and herbs, spices, and oil before adding it to the pan. You will find a number of delicious recipes for seitan on the Dukan Diet website (www.dukandiet.com).

Tempeh Of Indonesian origin, tempeh is made by fermenting soybeans. Tempeh has a firm texture and a natural nutty mushroom taste. It is rich in protein, with a low fat content and no cholesterol. It is a choice food for vegetarians.

A word of warning! Tempeh's carbohydrate content limits its place in my diet, where it can only be used as a tolerated food.

Soy or Vegetable Burgers Soy and vegetable burgers are useful essentially to vegetarians who do not eat meat. A very large variety of these products is sold by the large food retailers, but the disadvantage of this wide choice of brands and flavors is the mix of very different ingredients.

Some burgers are soy based, whereas others are based on cereals or on vegetables. This variety has a big impact on the nutritional composition.

It is essential to read the labels on these products, as the fat content can vary from single to double digits. It is also important to check the carbohydrate content, which is the limiting factor in my diet. I have selected two brands from among the most widely used products, Boca and MorningStar Farms.

From Boca, choose Boca Grilled Vegetable, Boca All American Flame Grilled, Boca Original Vegan, or Boca Cheeseburger. From MorningStar Farms, choose MorningStar Farms Classic Burger made with Organic Soy or MorningStar Farms Grillers.

Textured Soy Protein (TSP) Textured soy protein products are prepared using de-oiled soy flour that is mixed with water and heated under pressure. The mixture is then dried and broken up into granules or larger pieces.

Textured soy proteins have numerous advantages. They contain twice as much protein as beef. They are low in calories and do not contain cholesterol. They can be easily stored and can be kept for a very long time. Finally, they are very good value and easy to cook. Their texture is similar to meat, and they are designed to be hydrated and prepared in the same way as meat. In their raw state, they have a crunchy consistency and a hint of peanut flavor, which makes them very appealing as a snack.

A word of warning! In my diet, as is the case for tempeh, the carbohydrate content in TSP products means that they can only be used as a tolerated food.

Soy Milk Soy milk is a nondairy drink high in vegetable proteins and low in calories, carbohydrates, calcium, and vitamin D. It does not contain cholesterol.

Soy milk can be used as a milk substitute for individuals who do not drink cow's milk: vegetarians and people who are lactose-intolerant or do not like the taste of cow's milk or have a tendency toward high cholesterol.

Soy milk can be drunk plain or flavored and can be used to make all kinds of sauces usually based on milk, such as Béchamel.

A word of warning! Because of its carbohydrate content, you are limited to 2 glasses of unflavored soy milk per day, to replace nonfat cow's milk.

Soy yogurt Soy yogurt is made from soy milk and has the same characteristics. It offers an alternative to people who are lactose-intolerant, who have difficulty digesting dairy products, or who are pure vegans.

With regard to its nutritional and calorific value, soy yogurt is very similar to low-fat milk yogurt, with an average fat content of 2 percent depending on the brand, but cholesterol-free.

You are permitted two 6-ounce natural soy yogurts (no sugar) per day.

Category 9: Nonfat Dairy Products

Nonfat milk, nonfat yogurt, nonfat sour cream, nonfat cream cheese, and nonfat cottage cheese were developed to make losing weight easier. Just as the transformation of milk into cheese is responsible for the elimination of lactose, the only sugar found in milk, these fat-free dairy products contain practically nothing but protein, which is why they are so useful when we are looking for pure proteins during the Attack phase.

For some years now, milk producers have sold a new generation of yogurts sweetened with aspartame or Splenda or enriched with fruit pulp. While artificial sweeteners and other flavorings have no calorie content, the added fruit introduces unwanted carbohydrates. This drawback is compensated for by the fact that these gratifying treats give you the opportunity to enjoy a sweet and so can help you follow the overall diet program.

So that the following instructions are clear, there are three sorts of 0 percent fat yogurt: (1) natural yogurt; (2) flavored yogurts (e.g., coconut, vanilla, lemon); and (3) fruit yogurts, which have little bits of fruit or a fruit purée base.

- Natural and flavored yogurts are allowed without any restriction.
- Nonfat fruit yogurts are allowed, but no more than 8 ounces per day. However, if you want a lightning-fast start to your Attack phase diet, you are better off avoiding them altogether and even more so if you have hit a weight plateau.

Category 10: 1½ Quarts of Water per Day

As I have already told you, and at the risk of repeating myself, drinking 1½ quarts of water a day is indispensable and non-negotiable. Even if you are following the diet very carefully, if you do not thoroughly flush out your system, your weight loss will stop. The waste from your burning of fats will accumulate and extinguish the metabolic fire.

All types of water are allowed, including spring waters, as long as they do not contain too much sodium. If you do not like plain water, you can drink carbonated water, since carbonation has no effect on weight; it is only water high in sodium that must be avoided.

In addition, if you do not care for cold drinks, remember that tea, herbal tea, coffee, and any other hot drink are all assimilated as water and count toward your obligatory 1½ quarts of water per day.

Finally, diet drinks that do not have more than 1 calorie per 8 ounces are all allowed at every stage of the Dukan Diet. Nutritionists are divided when it comes to drinks sweetened with aspartame. Some think that the body detects and compensates for their trickery, whereas others think that their use provokes further cravings for sugar.

As far as I am concerned, my experience has taught me that abstaining from sugar, no matter for how long, never gets rid of the taste or the longing for sugar. So I see no reason to deprive yourself of this calorie-free treat. Furthermore, I have noticed that using these drinks make following the diet a lot easier and that their sweet flavor, strong smell, color, and bubbles, as well as their association with festivities and fun, all contribute to a powerful sensory gratification that soothes those cravings for "something else" that so often tempt those of us who like to snack.

This is the moment to talk about the controversy surrounding aspartame. To put it bluntly, some people are concerned that it may be carcinogenic, and I can understand why this is worrying. In my opinion, there is no need for all this controversy. Aspartame has been used as a sweetener by billions of individuals in every country in the world for twenty-five years without ever having given rise to any complaints or side effects and certainly not any human cancers. As far as I am concerned, I see no reason at all to deprive people on a diet who particularly like sweet tastes.

Category 11: 1½ Tablespoons of Oat Bran

For years, the first two actual weight loss phases in my program did not contain any starchy foods, cereals, or flour-based foods. The program worked fine without them, but many of the men and women who followed it eventually ended up longing for carbohydrates.

I discovered oat bran while attending a cardiology conference in America, where there was a presentation on how it reduces cholesterol and diabetes. I brought some home and one morning, having run out of flour, I created a special pancake, which I now call the Dukan Oat Bran Galette, for my daughter Maya. It is made of oat bran, an egg, and non-fat Greek yogurt sweetened with aspartame.

Maya loved it and felt completely full, so this spurred me on to suggest to my patients that they try the galette as well. Their enthusiasm for it persuaded me to include it in my method and my books. This is how oat bran gradually became a fundamental part of my method, the only carbohydrate allowed among the proteins and even within the sanctuary of the Attack phase. Why?

First, from a clinical perspective, I very quickly noticed an improvement in results: my patients followed the diet better over the long term; they felt less hungry and full sooner; and all in all, they were much less frustrated.

To try to understand how oat bran works, I looked at the studies available on it. Oat bran is the fibrous husk that surrounds and protects the oat grain. The grain, used to make rolled oats, is rich in simple sugars. Oat bran is the grain's jacket. It has few simple sugars but is very rich in proteins and particularly in soluble fibers. These fibers have two physical properties that give oat bran its therapeutic role.

On average, oat bran can absorb up to twenty-five times its volume of water. This means that as soon as it reaches the stomach, it swells and takes up enough space to very quickly make you feel full. It is also extremely high in soluble fiber and can reduce the absorption of dietary fat. Because oat bran makes you feel full and pushes food through your system more quickly, it is a precious ally in my battle against the weight problem epidemic.

I have done my own research on oat bran and have found that the way the bran is produced greatly determines how effective it is. Two manufacturing parameters, milling and sifting, are crucial. Milling involves grinding the bran and determines the size of its particles; sifting involves separating the bran from the oat flour. If the milling is too fine, the bran loses almost all its effectiveness. Likewise, if the bran is too coarse, its useful surface viscosity is lost. If the bran is not thoroughly sifted, it is not sufficiently pure and contains too much flour.

Ideally, milling should produce particles with a medium+ size (technically called M2bis). As for sifting, it is after it has been sifted for a sixth time, B6, that oat bran has negligible fast carbohydrate content. These two indexes together make up the overall M2bis-B6 index.

I am currently working with international manufacturers and distributors, sharing these results with them to try to get them to adopt the milling-sifting index, which makes production a little more expensive but produces a more nutritional bran. In the meantime, the recommended type of bran can be found on the Dukan Diet website, www .dukandiet.com.

During the Attack phase, I prescribe 1½ tablespoons of oat bran per day and recommend eating it as prepared in the Dukan Oat Bran Galette.

Dukan Oat Bran Galette

This light and easy pancake is a tasty way to eat your oat bran.

MAKES 1 GALETTE
Preparation time: 10 minutes

1 egg white

2 tablespoons oat bran

2 tablespoons fat-free plain Greek yogurt

1 teaspoon zero-calorie sweetener suited for cooking and
baking, such as Splenda, for a sweet pancake

or

Pepper, herbs, and/or chopped garlic for a savory pancake

In a small bowl, beat the egg white until foamy. In a separate bowl, combine the oat bran, Greek yogurt, and sweetener *or* seasonings. Add the beaten egg white and mix until blended.

Place a small nonstick pan over medium heat. Pour the pancake mixture into the pan and cook for around 5 minutes, or until the underside is golden and the upper side starts to dry. Flip the galette with a spatula and continue cooking the other side for an additional 5 minutes.

Remove to a plate and allow to cool briefly before serving.

Most of my patients eat their galette for breakfast to avoid feeling famished midmorning. Others eat the galette for lunch with a nice slice of smoked salmon or some thinly sliced ham or turkey breast. Other patients have the galette in late afternoon, at the "danger hour" when cravings can overtake them, or even after supper when they want to rummage around in the cupboard to find a final treat before bedtime. If you are going through a difficult period when irrepressible cravings are overwhelming, for a day or two (and I really do mean for only a day or two), you can eat more oat bran and up to three galettes per day.

Extras

Nonfat milk, either fresh, UHT, or powdered, is allowed and can improve the taste and the consistency of tea or coffee; it can also be used to make sauces, cream desserts, custard tarts, and many other dishes.

Sugar is not allowed, but aspartame and Splenda are perfectly acceptable and can be used without restriction, even by pregnant women.

Vinegar, spices, herbs, thyme, garlic, parsley, onion, and shallots are not only allowed but highly recommended. Using them brings out the flavor of foods and heightens their sensory value. These oral sensations trigger our nervous system, which is responsible for whether we feel full or not, contributing to our feeling of being satisfied. To be clear, I am saying quite simply that spices are not just taste enhancers, which in itself is no small achievement, but that they are foods that encourage weight loss.

What certain spices such as vanilla or cinnamon do is offer their warm and reassuring taste in exchange for sugary flavors. Others such as coriander, curry powder, and cloves can cut down the need for salt, especially for women who suffer from water retention and want to add salt to everything even before they have even tasted it.

Pickles (made without sugar), as well as pickled onions, are allowed, as long as they are condiments. If eaten in too large a quantity, they become a vegetable and outside the Attack phase's pure protein requirement.

Lemons can be used to flavor fish or seafood but cannot be consumed as lemon juice or lemonade, even without sugar, because although sour, lemons are still a source of sugar and are therefore incompatible with the program's first two phases, the Attack and Cruise phases.

Mustard and salt are acceptable but must be used in moderation. There are salt-free mustards and low-sodium diet salts if you want to use them liberally.

Ordinary ketchup is not allowed because it is both very salty and very sweet, but there are sugar-free natural ketchups that can be used in moderation and high-quality tomato purées and pastes that turn into a real treat with just a little flavoring and spicing up—without any of that sweet aftertaste that does not go well with meats.

Sugar-free chewing gum deserves better than this single entry in the extras category. To my mind, it is extremely useful in the fight against weight problems and especially so during my program's first two weight loss phases, the Attack and Cruise phases. I do not usually chew gum myself, as chewing is inelegant, but if I am overstressed, I do have some.

"Bruxism" is what dentists call the nighttime habit of grinding your teeth until the enamel is worn down. And as many overweight people often eat under stress, chewing gum can slow down this mechanical swing toward eating whenever you feel under pressure. What is more, a mouth that is busy chewing gum cannot take in or chew anything else, so this is a technique for keeping your mouth full. Many scientific studies have also proved at regular intervals how useful chewing sugar-free gum is when battling weight problems, diabetes, and even tooth decay.

Of course we are only talking here about so-called sugar-free gum. Select your sugar-free chewing gum according to taste but go for the ones whose flavor lasts longest in your mouth.

All oil is forbidden, except in the smallest quantities for greasing a frying pan. Even though olive oil justifiably has a reputation for protecting the heart and arteries, it is still oil, and pure fats have no place in a pure protein diet.

Apart from the allowable extras listed here and the food categories just described, you may eat *nothing else.* All other foods and drinks—anything that is not explicitly mentioned on this list—are forbidden during the Attack diet's relatively brief kick-start period.

Concentrate on what you are allowed to eat and forget the rest. Make sure you get enough variety and pick ingredients for your meals in any order you want so as to keep things interesting. And do not ever forget that all the foods allowed and on this list are for you, really and truly for you.

Some General Advice

Eat As Often As You Like

Do not forget that the secret of this diet is to eat a lot and to eat before hunger strikes so that you avoid succumbing to a tempting food not on the list.

Never Skip Meals

Skipping meals is a bad mistake that often stems from good intentions but that can, little by little, destabilize your diet. Whatever you save by not eating one meal you not only make up for by eating more at the next, but your body reverses this initial economy by increasing the "profit" it gets out of the next meal by extracting every last calorie. Furthermore, if you suppress and fuel your hunger, you will be driven toward more comforting foods, forcing you to rely increasingly on your willpower to resist, and eventually the strain will undermine even your best intentions.

Drink Whenever You Eat

For some strange reason, an outdated piece of advice from the 1970s not to drink at mealtimes still remains in the public mind. This advice can be harmful for those on a diet, particularly a pure protein diet, because not drinking at mealtimes may make you forget to drink at all. Drinking at mealtimes also increases gastric volume and makes you feel full and satisfied. Finally, water dilutes food and slows down its absorption so that you feel satiated for longer.

Do Not Run Out of the Foods You Need for Your Diet

Always have on hand a wide choice of the eleven food categories that are going to become your best friends. Take them with you whenever you go out.

Before You Eat Something, Check Whether It Is on the List

Just to be extra sure, keep this list with you during the first week. It is simple and can be summed up in a few words: lean meats, organ meats, poultry, lean ham, all fish and seafood, eggs, nonfat dairy products, and water.

Breakfast

Breakfast is an important meal in our pure protein diet. Coffee or tea, sweetened with aspartame or Splenda if you like, with or without nonfat milk, and enjoyed with a nonfat yogurt, boiled egg, a slice of turkey, or light ham is much better nutritionally than a pastry or chocolate-flavored cereal, and it is also more satisfying and stimulating.

Breakfast is the perfect time to cook your oat bran galette (see page 54). If you are in too much of a hurry to make the galette, you can eat the oat bran as a hot cereal by mixing 1 tablespoonful of oat bran with some hot nonfat milk sweetened with aspartame or Splenda, or mix it with yogurt to give it a thicker texture.

Take care! During this Attack phase, you must not exceed the daily dose of 1½ tablespoons of oat bran so as not to disrupt the specific action of the proteins.

Eating in Restaurants

With a little imagination, the pure protein diet is easy to follow. Fish, seafood, poultry, and meat generally come in many different guises. You should be able to find some that have been prepared without any fat. You may have to ask to have your dish served without the sauce. The difficulty comes afterward, when dessert fans are tempted to eat something sweet. The best strategy is to have a coffee, or you may find that some restaurants now serve low-fat and nonfat dairy products. Otherwise you can always have a nonfat yogurt or fruit yogurt in your car or at the office so that you can end your meal on a satisfying note.

How Long Should the Attack Phase Last?

How long to follow the Attack diet is one of the most important decisions in the Dukan Diet, because this pure protein attack is not only the kick start that gives you the initial impetus but also molds and sets the tone for the program on which the three other diet phases are based.

Proteins are extremely dense foods that remain present for a long time in the digestive system, making us feel full. As they are broken down during metabolism, ketones are produced, which are well known for creating a feeling of satiety. These two properties mean that proteins are useful for combating compulsive behavior and introducing order into unbalanced eating habits.

Finally, because the Attack diet is extremely effective, it produces obvious and immediate results, making you feel powerful and enthusiastic, and pumping up your motivation for the long-term haul. That is why it is so important to succeed in this first stage and to decide on its exact ideal duration.

On Average the Attack Phase Lasts 5 Days

This is the time the diet needs to produce its best results without encountering resistance from the body's metabolism and before the dieter becomes weary of it. This is also the attack period that best suits the sort of weight loss that most people want to achieve—that is, between 20 and 40 pounds.

For a Weight Loss Under 20 Pounds

A 3-day attack best suits this goal as it allows you to proceed effortlessly to the Cruise phase, which alternates days of pure protein with days of both proteins and vegetables.

For a Weight Loss Under 10 Pounds

If you would rather avoid an all-too-rapid start, a single day may be enough. This first day takes your body by surprise and produces a satisfying weight loss that is enough to encourage you to get started with the diet program.

For Serious Cases of Obesity

When the goal is to lose over 40 pounds, when motivation is really intense, or when previous experience with other diets has always resulted in the lost weight being regained, this phase may last 7 days or even as long as 10 days. An Attack diet of this length should only be begun after consulting with your doctor and on the express condition that you drink enough fluids throughout the entire Dukan Diet and especially the Attack phase.

How the Body Reacts During the Pure Protein Diet: The Surprise Effect and the Need to Adapt to a New Way of Eating

The first day of the Attack diet is one of adaptation and combat. While the door is open to many categories of popular and tasty foods, it is firmly closed to other categories that you may be in the habit of eating without thinking about just how many and the quantities you consume.

If you feel restricted (and the Attack phase can initially overwhelm the less motivated), the best remedy is to take full advantage of the diet's instructions to eat as much as you want of the permitted foods.

On the first day, eat more than you would normally. Make up for the foods you cannot eat with the quantity of the foods you can have. And, above all, organize yourself so that you always have all these essential foods available at all times.

Also, by drinking more water than you have ever drunk before, you will feel as if "there is something there" and more satisfied. You will need to go to the bathroom more often. The next morning, get on your scale, and you will be amazed by your first day's results.

Weigh yourself frequently, especially during the first three days. From one hour to the next, you could see new results. Get into the habit of weighing yourself every day of your life: Although for those who put on weight, the scale is an enemy, it is a friend and provides just reward for anyone who loses weight. Any weight loss, no matter how tiny, will be your very best incentive.

You Might Feel a Little Tired During the First 2 Days and Not Up to Prolonged Activity

This is not the right time to push your body to extremes. Avoid hard physical exercise, competitive sports, and, in particular, skiing at high altitudes. If you already do some gentle gymnastics, jogging, or swimming, keep this up but, whatever you do, make sure you walk for 20 minutes a day as this is an integral part of the program. As you will see in the chapter on exercise, these 20 minutes are not just recommended; they are prescribed, and this means they are non-negotiable.

By the third day, your tiredness should disappear and is usually replaced by a sense of euphoria and dynamic energy, which is further reinforced by the encouraging messages of your scales.

You Might Experience Bad Breath and a Dry Mouth

Bad breath and a dry mouth occur with any weight loss diet, but they will be more evident with the pure protein Attack diet. They are a sign that you are losing weight, and as such you should welcome them as proof of success. You can ease these symptoms by drinking more.

After the Fourth Day, You Can Expect Some Constipation

For people who are already prone to constipation and for those who do not drink enough, constipation at this stage of the diet is even more likely. For others, bowel movements may simply be less frequent, but do not take this as a sign of constipation. It is just a reduction in the amount of waste due to the low fiber content of proteins.

If this initial constipation bothers you, buy some wheat bran flakes and add 1 tablespoonful along with your oat bran to your galette or to your dairy products. Above all, drink as much as is recommended, because water not only makes you urinate, it also softens the stools, improving intestinal contractions and digestion.

More serious constipation is unpleasant, and you must do something about it. Your pharmacist can offer advice and may recommend some natural products based on fruit fiber. If these products are not enough, you need to see your doctor. Try to resist the temptation to take laxatives, which are too aggressive and to which you could eventually become habituated.

Your Hunger Will Disappear After the Third Day

You will find your hunger disappearing after the third day because of the increased release of ketones, the most powerful natural hunger suppressants. The monotony of eating all proteins these first few days has a marked effect on your appetite. Hunger pangs and cravings for sugar disappear completely. The quantity of protein you consume, considerable over these first days, gradually decreases.

Should You Take Vitamins?

I do recommend taking vitamins, but it is hardly compulsory for such a short period of only 3 to 5 days. On the other hand, if you need to follow the alternating protein diet for some time to deal with a major weight problem, it is a good idea to take a high-quality multivitamin. As soon as vegetables are allowed, you can have mixed salads with plenty of lettuce, raw peppers, tomatoes, carrots, and cucumbers—a natural source of various vitamins.

What Results Can You Expect from the Attack Diet?

The weight loss the pure protein diet produces is the most you could hope for in such a short period of time with a diet consisting of real food. It produces the same results as a powdered protein diet, or even total fasting, without any of their main drawbacks. Nevertheless, the weight loss depends on how many extra pounds you have at the outset. Obviously, someone who weighs over 200 pounds is going to shed those first pounds more quickly than someone just wanting to lose a few extra pounds before going on holiday.

Some people have also been "vaccinated" against dieting by their previous failures with other diets. Age is significant too. For women, hormones play an important role during puberty, after pregnancy, with oral contraception and—I cannot emphasize this too strongly—during menopause and postmenopause, peaking especially with any temporary or prolonged hormone therapy treatment.

With a 5-Day Pure Protein Attack Diet

Five days are generally the most popular and most effective time span, and usually the weight lost varies between 4 and 7 pounds. It may reach 8 or even 10 pounds for someone who is very overweight, especially an active man, or, at worst, it may only be 2 pounds for a menopausal woman on hormones who is prone to water retention and edema.

A woman's body retains water for 3 to 4 days before her period starts. This water retention reduces the elimination of waste and stops the combustion of fat, temporarily reducing the diet's effectiveness and blocking weight loss.

It is important to realize that in the days before a woman's period starts, the weight loss process has not been interrupted. It has just been camouflaged by water retention, and it will resume 2 or 3 days after the period is finished. If not properly explained and understood, this premenstrual plateau can make women despair, as they understandably think that all their efforts have been in vain, undermining their determination and prompting them to give the diet up.

So please, always wait until the end of your period before taking such a decision, because as soon as you eliminate the water, your low tide after the premenstrual high tide is when you often see the scales go down at a dizzying rate. If you have to get up to go to the bathroom several times in the course of one night, you might even lose 2 to 4 pounds.

With a 3-Day Attack Phase

If your Attack diet lasts just 3 days, you can expect to lose between 2 and 5 pounds.

With a Single, 1-Day Attack

If you follow the Attack diet for just 1 one day, you may lose around 2 pounds because the surprise effect is always greatest on the first day.

ATTACK PHASE SUMMARY

During the Attack phase, which can vary between 1 and 10 days depending on your circumstances, you have unlimited access to the food categories listed below.

From these categories you can eat all you want, without any restriction, at whatever time of day. Think of it as an all-day all-you-can-eat buffet. You are also free to mix and match these foods.

You can have everything on the list without exception. Everything that is not on the list is banned, so forget about those foods for the moment, knowing that very soon you will have them all again.

1. Lean meats: beef (except ribs and rib eye), veal, grilled or roasted without oil or fat, buffalo, and venison, except cuts used for braising or stewing
2. Organ meats: kidneys, liver, and tongue
3. All poultry, except duck and goose, but without the skin
4. Lean pork
5. All fish—fatty, lean, white, oily, raw or cooked
6. All shellfish
7. Low-fat ham, sliced low-fat chicken
8. Eggs

9. Nonfat dairy products
10. At least 1½ quarts of water or mineral water with a low salt content
11. The oat bran galette or 1½ tablespoons of oat bran added to nonfat milk or nonfat yogurt
12. A compulsory 20-minute walk per day
13. Extras: coffee, tea, vinegar, flavorings, spices, herbs, pickles, lemon (not lemonade), salt and mustard (in moderation)

Apart from these extras and the main food categories described, *eat nothing else.* Anything and everything that is not expressly mentioned on this list is forbidden during the relatively brief period of time that the Attack phase lasts.

Therefore, concentrate on everything you are allowed to have and forget the rest. Vary your meals, mix and match in whatever order, make your menus interesting, and never forget that you can have as much as you want of all the foods on this list.

THE
CRUISE
PHASE

The Alternating Protein Diet—
Protein + Vegetables

At the end of the Attack phase, the Dukan Diet is underway and the Cruise phase—what I call the alternating protein diet—begins, which will take you straight to your chosen weight.

This phase actually consists of two alternating diets: one day, the protein + vegetable diet and then the next day, the pure protein diet, and so on until you reach your target weight.

Having examined in detail how the pure protein Attack diet works, now let's look at the protein + vegetable diet.

Here again, as with the Attack phase, there is not a standard version of the alternating rhythm of the two diets for everyone. Rather, the rhythm is adapted to each person and situation based on the factors that I will describe shortly.

For a long time, the rhythm I used most frequently was the 5/5 alternating rhythm, 5 days of proteins + vegetables alternating with 4 days of pure proteins. With time, and especially for people wanting to lose over 20 pounds, I have slowly come round to the 1/1 alternating rhythm with a single day of proteins + vegetables followed by a single day of pure proteins. My own statistics showed that at the end of the first month, the weight loss for both groups was the same, but more decisively, over the long term, the risk of tiring of the 5/5 alternating rhythm was greater than for the 1/1 one.

In my experience, the majority of dieters have always gone for the most radical solutions, such as 7 to 10 days of the Attack diet and then the 5/5 alternating rhythm. This confirms one of my most consistent observations as a practitioner: that when overweight individuals who have resisted the idea of dieting for a long time feel motivated to suddenly start dieting, they know perfectly well that the force that has suddenly taken them over is as powerful as it is fragile, and that the best way to maintain it is to follow as closely as possible instructions that are precise, simple, focused, concrete, and non-negotiable. For this reason, I am asking you to trust me and to follow this Cruise phase using the 1/1 alternating rhythm.

By the time you finish the protein-only Attack diet, especially after 5 days, you really start to miss one particular food category—vegetables, raw or cooked—which is great because this is just the right time to introduce them.

Everything that was allowed in the pure protein diet is still allowed, with the same freedom of quantity, time of day, and combinations. Just do not make the mistake of eating only vegetables and no proteins.

Vegetables You Can and Cannot Eat

From now on, as well as protein-rich foods, you are allowed all cooked or raw vegetables and, here again, without restriction regarding quantity, time of day, or combination.

You can eat tomatoes, cucumbers, radishes, spinach, asparagus, leeks, green beans, cabbage, mushrooms, celery, fennel, all types of lettuce, eggplant, zucchini, summer squash, peppers, and, provided you do not have them at every meal, carrots and beets.

Vegetables considered to be starchy foods are, however, forbidden: potatoes, corn, fresh or dried peas, beans, and lentils. Avocado is also forbidden; it is not a vegetable, but a fruit, and a very fatty fruit in the bargain. Rice, quinoa, barley, wheat berries, millet, and other grains are not allowed.

How Should These Vegetables Be Prepared?

You can eat these vegetables raw or cooked. However, if you can digest raw vegetables, it is always preferable to eat vegetables when they are fresh and uncooked so you do not lose any of the vitamins they contain.

The Problem with Dressings

Dressings may appear harmless, but they are a major problem for weight loss diets. Indeed, many people base their diet around salads and crudités, which are low in calories and rich in fiber and vitamins. This is perfectly true, but do not forget that it is the salad dressing that upsets the balance of these good qualities. Let's take a simple example: in an ordinary salad bowl containing two heads of lettuce and 2 tablespoons of oil, the salad accounts for 20 calories and the oil for 200 calories, which is why so many diets based on mixed salads fail.

We also need to clear up the ambiguity concerning olive oil. Even though this symbol of the Mediterranean lifestyle is recognized as protecting us against cardiovascular disease, it is no less rich in calories than any other oil on the market.

For these reasons, during the first two actual weight loss phases, the Attack and Cruise phases, it is crucial that you avoid preparing green vegetables, cooked or raw, with a sauce or dressing that contains more than 1 teaspoon of vegetable oil.

Basic Vinaigrette 1

This easy, flavorful vinaigrette uses a tiny amount of oil.

1 tablespoon mustard (Dijon or, even better, French whole-grain
    mustard)
5 tablespoons balsamic vinegar
1 teaspoon vegetable oil
Salt and freshly ground black pepper to taste
Optional:
1 large garlic clove
7 or 8 basil leaves

Take a clean, empty jar and add the mustard, balsamic vinegar, vegetable oil, salt, and freshly ground black pepper. If you like garlic, add a large clove to marinate in the bottom of the jar, together with 7 or 8 basil leaves. Cover the jar and shake vigorously to mix the dressing before serving.

Variation:

If you do not like balsamic vinegar, you can select another one. Just use a little less: 4 tablespoons for wine, sherry, or raspberry vinegar; 3 tablespoons for champagne vinegar.

Vinegar is a condiment that can play a major role in any diet. An interesting paradox has recently been discovered: that humans can distinguish four universal flavors—sweet, salty, bitter, and sour—yet vinegar is the only substance in the human food list to provide that precious and rare sour taste.

What is more, recent studies have also demonstrated the impact that oral sensation—the quantity and the variety of flavors—has on producing the feeling of satisfaction and fullness. For example, we know today that the taste of certain spices, such as cloves, ginger, turmeric, star anise, and cardamom, work on the hypothalamus, the area in our brain that measures these sensations until the feeling of satiety is triggered. So it is very important to use as wide a range of spices as possible, and as much as possible, preferably at the start of a meal, and, if you are not already a great fan, to try to get used to them.

Yogurt Dressing

This dressing, made with nonfat yogurt, makes an easy savory sauce.

6 to 8 ounces nonfat plain yogurt
1 tablespoon mustard (Dijon, if possible)
Dash of vinegar
Salt, pepper, and herbs to taste

Beat the yogurt and mustard together until it has the consistency of mayonnaise. Add the vinegar, salt, pepper, and herbs.

Vegetables as a Cooked Garnish

Now is your chance to use green beans, spinach, leeks, cabbages of all varieties, mushrooms, braised greens, fennel, and celery. These vegetables can be cooked in water, boiled, or, even better, steamed to retain the maximum amount of vitamins. You can also bake them in the oven in the juice from your meat or fish.

Finally, cooking *en papillote* (literally, "in parchment paper," but aluminum foil can also be used) combines all the advantages as far as nutrition and taste are concerned; it is particularly suitable for preparing fish, in particular salmon, which remains tender when cooked on a bed of leeks or eggplant.

Introducing vegetables after the pure protein phase brings freshness and variety to the initial Attack diet. Things are easier, even comfortable. Now it is practical to start a meal off with a salad, well seasoned and rich in color and flavor; or, in winter, with a soup, followed by a meat or fish dish gently stewed with flavorful and fragrant vegetables.

How Many Vegetables Are You Allowed?

In principle, quantity is not limited. But it is wise not to go beyond common sense simply to take advantage of the fact that you are not restricted. I know patients who eat huge mixed salads without even feeling hungry, chomping through their meal as if they had a mouth full of chewing gum. Eat until you no longer feel hungry, but do not keep going. This does not alter the rule that quantities are unrestricted, which is at the heart of my program.

Whatever quantity you eat, you will still lose weight, but at a slower and less encouraging rate.

I want to tell you about a frequent reaction to the changeover from the strictly protein Attack diet to the diet now enhanced by the introduction of vegetables.

Very often, weight loss is spectacular during the first phase and then, when vegetables are introduced, the scales seem to get stuck and do not go down, or may even show a slight increase in pounds. Do not worry—you are not slipping backward. So what is happening?

During the Attack phase, eating only proteins has a powerful diuretic effect. Reserve fat is lost, as well as a large quantity of water that had been stagnating in the body for a long time. This combination of eliminated water and fat explains why your scales show an impressive loss.

But when vegetables are added to proteins, water is retained once more, which explains the weight plateau. The real weight loss continues, but it is being camouflaged by the return of water. Be patient, and as soon as the pure protein days return, the loss of water weight will start again, and you will see how many pounds you have really lost.

You must realize, however, that this is going to be your way of life during this period of alternating diets until you reach your target weight. It is always going to be the pure protein days that get the machine moving and that are responsible for the diet's overall effectiveness. So do not be surprised to see your weight go down at regular intervals. The weight loss levels out during the vegetable days and then drops down to another level during the pure protein days, and so on.

A Choice of Alternating Rhythms

The diet of alternating proteins, building on the momentum and speed generated by the pure protein Attack diet, is now responsible for guiding you to your chosen goal. This phase will occupy the largest part of the strictly weight loss period of the Dukan Diet.

The rhythmical addition of vegetables greatly reduces the pure proteins' impact and gives this entire second phase in the diet a kind of syncopated pace, both for organizing your meals and for the results obtained. Thus there will be pauses interrupted by accelerations, a series of conquests followed by resting periods, all leading in alternate sequence, nevertheless, to your end goal.

What rhythm should this diet take? I will sum it up briefly:

- *In the short term, the most effective rhythm is 5/5:* 5 days of pure proteins followed by 5 days of proteins + vegetables. This is not the easiest rhythm: it does start off spectacularly, but it slows down and may become burdensome.
- *The other solution is the 1/1 rhythm:* 1 day of pure proteins followed by 1 day of vegetables + proteins. This alternating rhythm takes longer to get going, but in 20 days it will have caught up, and over the long term it is easier to follow and generates less frustration.
- *There is a third way, which is suitable if you only have a little weight to lose, the 2/7 rhythm:* 2 days of pure proteins on Mondays and Thursdays and 5 days of proteins + vegetables during the rest of the week.
- *Finally, there is a variation on the 2/7 rhythm—the 2/0 rhythm:* 2 days of pure proteins per week, on Mondays and Thursdays, followed by 5 days of no particular diet but avoiding any extremes. This is the diet that best suits some women with cellulite, who are slim on top but heavy around the hips and the thighs especially.

Some Additions for the Cruise Phase

Oat Bran

During the Cruise phase, the amount of oat bran you should eat is increased from the 1½ tablespoons per day of the Attack phase to 2 tablespoons per day, prepared in the same way as for the Attack phase.

Exercise

Similarly, the recommended exercise is increased from the 20-minute walk of the Attack phase to a 30-minute walk in the Cruise phase. If you are on a stagnation plateau, increase this to a 60-minute walk for 4 days, just until you break through this plateau.

How Much Weight Can You Expect to Lose?

If you are significantly overweight, by 40 pounds or more, the loss is difficult to predict week by week, but experience has shown that one can expect to lose around 2 pounds a week.

During the first half of the Cruise phase, when you can expect a weight loss of 3 to 4 pounds per week, you can potentially lose the first 20 pounds in approximately 2 months.

Beyond the first 2 months, the curve decreases progressively because of a metabolic defense mechanism that I will explain in further detail when we come to the Consolidation phase, the third stage of the program. The curve then flattens at just over 2 pounds per week before dipping below 2 pounds a week, with odd periods of stagnation for women with premenstrual syndrome or if there is any bingeing.

On this subject, you need to know that the body puts up little resistance to the loss of the first few pounds. It has a greater reaction when the plundering of its fat reserves becomes more threatening. In theory, this would be just the moment to step up your diet. But in practice, the very opposite often occurs. The strongest willpower sometimes weakens in the face of long-suppressed temptations, and invitations to eat out that were once declined are now accepted.

But the real threat comes from elsewhere. The loss of the first 20 pounds brings general visible improvement: shape and suppleness return, breathlessness disappears, compliments come by the dozen, and you have the satisfaction of getting back into clothes that did not fit before. Add to all this the classic excuse of "just this once," and your wonderful strong determination from the early days suddenly makes way for bingeing followed by a return to drastic dieting, creating a chaotic, yo-yoing situation that soon becomes dangerous.

It is in such circumstances that—victorious up until now—you risk resting on your laurels and ending, up abandoning your goal. You have to realize that in the middle of the race, crossing the dangerous territory of weariness and self-satisfaction that is part of any prolonged diet, half of all dieters fall into this trap and let everything slip away.

In this event, there are three ways to react:

1. You can abandon the diet, sink into complacency and succumb to compulsive behavior patterns, but with a deep sense of failure that leads to your quickly putting the pounds back on, often going far beyond the weight you started out with.

2. Or, you can get back on track by resuming the Attack diet and sticking with it until your set goal is attained.

3. Or, you can admit that you feel incapable of going any further, but that you are ready to do whatever it takes to preserve what you have achieved so far. If this is your choice, stop the weight loss phase of the Dukan Diet and go directly to the Consolidation phase (see page 80). The Consolidation phase has a much more varied choice of food, and it is easy to work out how long it lasts (5 days for every pound you have lost). Then go to the Stabilization phase, in which you are allowed a completely free choice of food, with just 1 day per week of the pure protein diet.

How Long Should the Alternating Protein Diet Last?

The Cruise phase is the key time in the weight loss period, the one which will take you to your goal, your True Weight.

If you have over 40 pounds to lose, and if there are no other particular difficulties involved, you might hope to shed that weight over 20 weeks of the alternating protein diet—that is, in a little under 5 months.

Resistant Cases

For some, however, losing weight may be more difficult for several reasons:

- For physiological reasons, such as a family tendency to obesity
- For psychological reasons, such as little self-discipline or weak motivation
- For individuals with a history of having dieted many times with bad diets or diets not followed properly or simply abandoned midway.
- For girls during prepuberty, and for women when their periods are irregular, or during pregnancy, and above all during perimenopause and menopause

In all these cases, weight loss will be slowed down and will require specific adjustments. Even so, even in difficult cases, the spirit of the Attack phase is so strong, and the pace of the first 2 or 3 weeks of the Dukan Diet so intense, that most resistance and inhibitions are overcome, resulting generally in an initial loss of 8 to 10 pounds. This is the point at which old demons can reappear to slow things down.

If You Are Predisposed to Being Excessively Overweight

If your family history predisposes you to being obese, in less than a month you will likely fall under the threshold of losing 2 pounds a week and reach an acceptable pace of 6 to 7 pounds a month for 2 to 3 months. This, added to your initial loss, will bring you to a loss of about 30 pounds. At this stage, your monthly weight loss will be further reduced to around 4 or perhaps 3 pounds a month.

You may then ask yourself, Is this all worth it? More often than not, the answer is no.

Unless you have been advised by your doctor to continue the weight loss part of the diet for reasons such as the threat of diabetes or severe and inoperable arthritis, or unless you have an imperative personal reason for doing so, it is probably best to stop the Cruise phase and not run the risk of undermining the results you've obtained so far. Instead you can go on to the Consolidation and Stabilization phases and can wait for better days to continue your weight loss to your original goal.

You can be proud of having lost around 35 pounds lost during your 4 months or so of following the alternating protein diet.

If You Are Not Very Motivated or Lack Willpower

If you are not very motivated or lack the willpower to follow the diet, you are in a worse position. You will also lose the first 8 to 10 pounds, but the temptation to give up will rear its head straightaway. In the best-case scenario, if you can count on those around you and can count on your doctor's helping you, you can expect to lose another 10 pounds in 5 weeks and then quickly go on to the Consolidation phase and even more quickly to the Stabilization phase, where you will have to agree to eat only proteins for 1 day a week for the rest of your life. You have to accept this painless and simple measure before you even start this program.

Overall result: 22 pounds in 2½ months using the alternating protein diet.

If Your Body Has Developed a Resistance to Dieting Because You Followed Poor Diets Badly in the Past

If your body has developed a resistance to dieting because you followed poor diets badly in the past, the Dukan Diet is your best selection. The Attack phase acts like a bulldozer, pushing aside all resistance. You, too, will lose 12 pounds during the first 3 weeks, but if you follow the Cruise phase instructions precisely, you will also continue to lose weight without interruption until you actually lose almost 45 pounds in 6 months on the alternating protein diet. And if you regain some of the weight you have lost, you can always return to the Attack phase later without any risk of developing resistance.

If You Are in Perimenopause or Menopause

If you are in perimenopause or menopause, you are facing that time in your life when you are most at risk of putting on weight, and especially so if you already have some extra pounds. Even losing the first few pounds in the Attack phase is a major undertaking. That is why it is vital for you to get your hormone balance under control before starting this program. Doing so is a matter for the gynecologist or family doctor.

Keep in mind that weight gained during menopause is not irreversible, though it is a difficult period to go through. You will, if armed and ready, get past this difficult stage in 6 months to a year. Well-managed hormone replacement therapy will give you the best basis for losing weight effectively. Without supervised hormone therapy, it can take up to a year to lose around 45 pounds.

Please Take Note!

If by following my program, you reach this point on your road map, you will have achieved your True Weight—well done.

However, going by my statistics, it is my duty to tell you that:

- 50 percent of readers stop here; they consider themselves cured. They forget that there are still two other phases to finish to ensure that their new weight is maintained over the long term. All those who are impatient will, without exception, put the weight back on or get caught up in eating patterns that can only end in failure. So you have been warned.

- The other 50 percent of my readers do not stop here but rather follow me into the Consolidation phase; 85 percent of these go right to the end. This is better, but not good enough.

- Only those who go on into the fourth and final Permanent Stabilization phase, and follow it, achieve the single goal that counts: being cured of being overweight.

- I hope with all my heart, dear reader, that you will not stop here and that you will continue to the very end of our joint undertaking. Otherwise I will have done what other diets have done for the past sixty years: I will have brought you with me into the desert and abandoned you just before you reach the oasis.

CRUISE DIET SUMMARY

Keep eating all the Attack diet foods and add the following vegetables, raw or cooked, without restricting quantities, combinations, or time of day: tomatoes, cucumbers, radishes, spinach, asparagus, leeks, string beans, cabbage, mushrooms, celery, fennel, Swiss chard, eggplant, zucchini, summer squash, peppers, and all salad greens, including chicory. You can even include carrots, beets, and artichokes, provided you do not eat them at every meal. These three vegetables contain a little more sugar than the others allowed in the alternating protein diet, but you can eat them liberally while you're losing weight at a normal rate. However, if your weight loss slows or you reach a plateau, reduce or eliminate their consumption until your weight loss resumes.

Throughout this Cruise phase, you will alternate periods of proteins with vegetables with periods without any vegetables until you reach your desired weight.

THE CONSOLIDATION PHASE

The Transition Diet

You have now arrived at your True Weight, or at the weight you considered acceptable and set as your goal at the start—or at a weight you want to settle for as acceptable or a half victory, because you know that the effort involved in going further is too much and risks jeopardizing what you have achieved so far.

The time of rigorous constraints is over, and you are at last on flat terrain. You and your body have made a prolonged effort, and you have been rewarded. But to rest on your laurels now is very dangerous. You have reached a weight that suits you, but this weight that you have achieved does not really quite belong to you yet. Get rid of the illusion that you have at last finally taken care of your weight problem and can now go back to your old ways. That would be catastrophic, because in no time at all you will be back to your old weight. I do not mean that you have to continue forever with the aggressive diet that you have just followed. Who would agree to that?

The extra pounds that made you follow this diet in the first place, especially if they were a substantial—or worse, a recurring—problem, were certainly no accident. Whether these pounds were due to your genes or were an acquired habit, there is something written inside you, a bit like the information on a hard disk, that will not disappear.

There is a way of keeping your new weight, and it will be the theme of the fourth phase of the program, the Permanent Stabilization phase. But you are not there yet because you are still predisposed to gain weight, and this tendency is now actually heightened by your body's defense impulse, as it thinks that it has been robbed of its reserves.

What you need to do is to make peace with your body, which is just waiting for the opportunity to replenish those reserves. This is the objective of this next phase—the Consolidation phase in which you consolidate the weight lost and which, when completed, will open the door to every dieter's dream: permanent weight stabilization at little cost.

But to be completely ready to start this Consolidation phase, you must understand why you are still too vulnerable, and your body too prone to weight rebound, for you to move straight to the Permanent Stabilization phase. After this brief but vital theoretical introduction, I will explain to you in detail how to follow this Consolidation phase in practice, the new foods it involves, and how long it lasts.

The Weight Rebound Reaction

When a body has lost a good number of pounds through effective dieting, several reactions conspire to put the weight back on. To understand them, you need to know that the buildup of fat reserves means that the body has surplus calories available in case of any future food shortage.

Fat was the simple solution nature came up with to conserve and store energy; it is the most concentrated form known in the animal kingdom (1 gram of fat = 9 calories). Nowadays, when food is completely and easily accessible, we may well ask ourselves what use storing fat is to our bodies.

But, again, you have to remember that our biological system was not designed for the modern world; it came into being at a time when access to food was hazardous and unpredictable and required struggle and hard work. Being fat was a precious survival tool for the first humans. The human body, whose biological programming has remained unchanged, still bestows the same importance on what it considers as its vital reserves and does not like to see them being plundered.

A body that is losing weight risks being left with no resources if there is the slightest interruption in its food supply. That is why it reacts—because it feels threatened biologically. All its reactions have one sole objective: to recover all the fat it has lost as soon as possible. Your body has three very effective ways of doing this:

- The first is to trigger hunger pangs and sharpen your appetite to encourage you to eat more; the more unsatisfying your previous diet was before you embarked on the Dukan Diet, the stronger this reaction will be.

- Your body's second strategy is to reduce its energy consumption. If you earn less money, you tend to spend less. Biological organisms react in a similar way. This is why many people complain about feeling cold during weight loss diets; your body is using less energy to keep you warm.

  The same goes for tiredness: when we feel tired, we avoid any unnecessary effort, excessive activity becomes difficult, and everything slows down. Memory and intellectual effort, which require a lot of energy, are also affected. The need for sleep and rest, which save energy, also increases. Hair and nails grow less rapidly. In short, in order to adapt to a long period of losing weight, the body goes into a kind of hibernation.

- Finally, the body's third reaction is the most efficient and the most dangerous one, whether you are trying to lose weight or are already stabilizing, as it consists in assimilating the calories from your food more efficiently. An individual who ordinarily gets 100 calories from a slice of bread will end up, at the end of the diet, assimilating 120 to 130 calories from the same slice. Each morsel is sifted through, and everything possible is absorbed. This increase in calorie extraction takes place in the small intestine.

Increase in appetite, reduction in energy used, and maximum extraction of calories consumed all combine to transform the overweight body that has just lost weight into a calorie sponge. This is usually the moment when you are so happy with your results that you assume you can lower your guard and return to your old habits. This is the most frequent and natural cause for those pounds quickly piling back on again.

So, after you have carefully followed a diet and attained your desired weight, this is the time to be most careful. It is called the rebound period; like a ball that has just touched the ground, weight has a tendency to bounce back.

How Long Does the Rebound Period Last?

There is still no natural or therapeutic method today to counter rebound. The best way to protect yourself against it is to know how long it will last so that during this time you can fight it with the correct eating strategy. Over time I have observed rebound effects in my patients and have concluded that the high-risk period for regaining weight lasts about 5 days for every pound lost—for example, 30 days for 6 to 7 pounds lost, or 100 days for 18 to 20 pounds lost.

I attach great importance to this rule because, here again, it is the lack of precise information that puts you at greatest risk when you have lost weight and finished dieting. Understanding the dangers and how long they last really helps you to get through the Consolidation phase and also to more easily accept the additional but crucial effort you will need to make to neutralize the rebound.

The simple passage of time during the Consolidation phase allows your system, which is on alert to conserve weight, to settle down and relax. Here my Stabilization diet awaits, with its three simple, concrete, and painless measures, including protein Thursdays.

Meanwhile, you must follow a new, more open Transition diet that offers freedom within limits. It is not a weight loss diet, but it is not yet a diet free from all constraints.

How Do You Choose Your Correct Stabilization Weight?

It is hard to maintain your new weight—even if you are set on doing everything you can to never regain the pounds you have fought so hard to lose—without having a precise weight target and without having defined a future weight objective that is both satisfying and realistic. I have witnessed too many failures, due in the most part to an unrealistic choice of stabilization weight.

Many formulas exist to define a person's ideal weight according to height, age, gender, and bone structure. All these formulas are theoretically applicable, but I am wary of them because they are about statistical individuals who in reality do not exist.

So, in place of a theoretical ideal weight, I tend to use the more realistic notion of a weight at which you can comfortably stabilize. The best way to calculate a good stabilization weight is to ask yourself what weight you can most easily achieve and at which you will feel good. There are two reasons for basing your stabilization weight on these factors.

Every mammal, including man, is biologically programmed to store as fat excess food consumed and not used. This fat is a strategic energy reserve necessary for survival when food is scarce. Today we live in a land of plenty and our problem is not finding food, but refusing it. However, your body's programming to store fat in case of a food shortage has remained the same.

As you lose weight, your body goes into alert mode, trying to protect its fat reserves. It becomes more efficient at using the food you give it so weight loss slows. At this point, you reach what I call a plateau of stagnation.

Trying to stabilize your weight when it has plateaued is doomed to fail, because the effort required is disproportionate to the result obtained. If you try anyway, it would require so much effort it would be unbearable in the long run.

Furthermore, please know that for people who were substantially overweight to start with, I place far greater emphasis on well-being than on the symbolic value of an abstract and supposedly "normal" weight. If you are predisposed to being overweight, you are not just "the average person," and you should not set a goal that does not suit who you are. What you need is to be able to live normally and happily; not burdened by the stress of an unrealistic goal. Stabilizing at this weight will be a remarkable feat in itself.

Finally, you have to bear in mind the maximum and minimum weights you have reached in all your weight fluctuations over the years, because no matter how long your maximum weight lasted, it is that weight your body will have forever recorded in its biological memory.

As an example of what I mean by the effect of your body's biological memory, let's imagine a woman 5 feet 6 inches tall who has, on just one day of her life, weighed over 210 pounds. It is an absolute impossibility that such a woman could ever hope to stabilize at around 112 pounds, as some theoretical tables suggest. Her body retains the biological memory of her maximum weight, and this memory can never be erased. To recommend that she stabilize her weight at 150 pounds is more sensible, at least on paper—but only if she already feels comfortable at that weight.

Another common mistake is that many dieters—ones who are very overweight as well as ones who are not quite so overweight—think that it will be easier to stabilize at a certain weight if they lose a little more so that they have a few pounds as a safety margin. However, wanting, for example, to go down to 125 pounds in order to stabilize at 150 pounds is not just an error, it is a huge mistake, because the amount of willpower wasted getting your weight down to 125 pounds will be sorely missed when you need it later in order to stabilize. The more you force your weight down, the more your system will be prone to rebound upward.

In conclusion, you must choose a weight that is achievable, high enough to be attainable and low enough to provide the gratification and well-being you will need to stick to that weight.

I call this weight the True Weight. It is not the same thing as the body mass index (BMI) (see page 116), which is useful for pinpointing high-risk groups but less useful for determining particular individual's weight and setting strategic goals.

How Do You Work Out Your True Weight?

By definition, each person's True Weight is personal. For starters, it must take a person's age and gender into account. For example, we know that with each decade, a woman's stable weight needs to be increased by 1.8 pounds and a man's by 2.6 pounds. Furthermore, a person's needs, and especially the likelihood of achieving a certain weight, will differ between age 20 and age 50.

When working out this True Weight, family history must also be considered. Here again, there is no point asking a woman whose family has a history of obesity to aim for the same stable weight as a woman whose family is by nature slim. In addition, it is absolutely essential to include the history of a person's weight problems, the crucial moment when weight started to get out of control: was it childhood, adolescence, or at a time of major stress, medical treatment, or depression—or for a woman, at her first contraceptive pill, with pregnancy, or in perimenopause? Each person is different from the next, and these differences need to be taken into consideration.

It is also equally necessary to take into account what I call the "weight range"—the difference between the least someone has ever weighed after the age of twenty and the most the person has weighed apart from during pregnancy. This range tells us what is recorded in that person's biological memory and remains there forever.

Also figuring into calculating a person's True Weight is how many unsuccessful diets have been followed, and which ones, as there are some diets from which the body never quite recovers—diets that go against nature and trigger "body anxieties." The best known of these diets are based on powdered or liquid meal substitutes, which are the very opposite of what is natural for humans to eat.

We are not programmed to feed on meal substitutes, and our bodies may develop a sort of adverse reaction that unfortunately makes us resistant to other diets. Fasting is a disaster for our muscle mass, because with fasting, the body has to use muscle to get the vital proteins it needs for its survival. But fasting is infinitely more natural than eating these meal substitutes, as it can happen in nature that a predator catches no prey and is forced to fast for a few days.

You can see that there are many different parameters used to calculate a person's True Weight and that it is too complex to be calculated just by using pen and paper. I recommend that you go to the Dukan Diet website (www.dukandiet.com), where you will find a free questionnaire with eleven questions that will let you find your True Weight. Answer them, and you will have your True Weight straightaway. Then you will know the exact bull's-eye for your target. You can measure the distance, I will give you the bow and arrow, and you will stand a much better chance of scoring a hit.

The Transition Diet Day by Day

You have just ended your final day of the alternating protein diet, and for the first time on your scales you have seen your True Weight, the weight that I hope you have managed to achieve. If this is not the case, then the weight that you set yourself when you started your diet. Like many others before you, carried away by your success, you feel tempted to continue to try and lose a little more to have a safety margin. Please do not think of doing this. The dice have been thrown, you wanted this weight, you have it, and now you have to summon all your strength to try and keep it. I am not just saying this: one in every two failures occurs in the 3 months after the desired weight has been attained.

How Long Should the Transition Diet Last?

The length of this transition diet is based on how much weight you have lost: 5 days on this new diet for every pound lost. For example:

If you have just lost 40 pounds, you must follow the transition diet for 40 × 5 days, or 200 days (6 months and 20 days). If you have lost 20 pounds, you will need to follow the diet for 100 days. Everyone can easily calculate the exact amount of time needed until the definitive Permanent Stabilization phase begins.

Am I going to give you the Permanent Stabilization diet at this point? No. You now realize that you are too vulnerable, you are like a deep-sea diver coming up from the depths who has to do it in stages for safety's sake. This is the role of the diet that I am now going to introduce.

During this Consolidation phase, you will follow as faithfully as possible the following transition diet, on which you can eat as much as you want from the foods I will outline below.

Proteins and Vegetables

Up to this point, during your Cruise phase, you alternated between proteins and proteins + vegetables. From now on, you do not have to alternate. You can eat all proteins and vegetables together and still have as much as you want.

Proteins and vegetables constitute a stable foundation on which you will build the Consolidation phase, as well as the final and Permanent Stabilization phase that will follow it. You can see why these two major food categories are so important, because for the rest of your life you can eat them without there being any limit on quantity, time of day, or combination.

You probably know all the foods by now, but I will briefly review them so as to avoid any misunderstanding. For more details, you will find the complete list in the chapters on the Attack phase and the Cruise phase. These allowed foods are

- Lean meats—the least fatty cuts of beef and veal, buffalo, and venison
- Organ meats such as liver, tongues, and kidneys
- Fish and seafood

- Poultry (except duck and goose), always without the skin
- Low-fat ham, sliced low-fat chicken and turkey
- Eggs
- Nonfat dairy products
- Raw and cooked vegetables
- 1½ quarts of water

As well as the above base of proteins and vegetables, the Consolidation phase introduces new foods that will improve your daily eating. They can be added in the following proportions and quantities.

One Serving of Fruit per Day

I'm sure most of you believe that fruit belongs to the "as much as you want" category because it is so naturally healthy. This is partly true: fruit is a natural product and it is also one of the best-known sources of vitamin C and carotene.

Fruit in its natural state was a colorful and satisfying reward for humans. It is only through intensive farming and selection that we nowadays have the impression that fruit is easy to come by. As it is, most fruit with a high sugar content, such as pineapples, bananas, and mangos, comes to us from tropical regions and was only recently introduced into our regular diet, thanks to progress in transportation.

In fact, fruit is not the prototype of a healthy and natural food. It is the only natural food that contains what diabetes specialists call rapid-assimilation sugars. Consumed in large quantities it can be unhealthy, especially for diabetics and overweight people who tend to eat fruit outside of mealtimes.

Rationed to 1 serving of fruit per day, you are now allowed to eat all types of fruit *except* bananas, grapes, cherries, dried fruits, and nuts (walnuts, peanuts, almonds, pistachios, macadamias, and cashews).

How much is a serving? With fruits the size of an apple, pear, orange, grapefruit, peach, or nectarine, a serving is 1 medium-size piece of fruit. For smaller fruits, or larger ones, use a normal serving: a cup of strawberries or raspberries, half of a medium cantaloupe or a quarter of a honeydew melon, an inch-thick slice of watermelon, 2 kiwis, 2 nice apricots, 1 small mango or half a large one. You can eat all these fruits, but remember, only 1 serving per day and not per meal.

Bear in mind that the best fruits for stabilizing your weight are the following, in descending order:

- Apples. I give priority to the apple, because its high pectin content helps keep you feeling full.
- Strawberries and raspberries. These are low in calories and look colorful and festive.
- Melon and watermelon, if you stick to the serving size, because of their high water and low calorie content.
- Grapefruit, for its pulp, is rich in pectin and low in calories.
- Kiwi is high in vitamin C and low in sugar content. Peaches and nectarines are full of flavor, with a luscious texture and moderate sugar content. Mango is the richest in vitamins A, C, and E, three major antioxidants.

Two Slices of 100 Percent Whole Grain Bread per Day

If you are prone to putting on weight, get into the habit of avoiding white bread. White flour is too refined, and like white and other simple sugars, it enters into the bloodstream too quickly and in too great a quantity.

One hundred percent whole grain bread tastes good and has a natural proportion of bran, which is a major ally in normal elimination.

For this Consolidation phase of the diet, you are still under strict surveillance as your body is waiting to extract calories from everything. But once you reach the Permanent Stabilization phase, you will be able to eat bread normally, as long as it is whole grain or, even better, enriched with bran or fiber. From now on, if you enjoy bread at breakfast, you may lightly spread your 2 slices of whole grain bread with some reduced-fat butter or spread. But you may also decide to eat these 2 slices of bread at some other time of the day, for a cold meat or ham sandwich at lunchtime, or in the evening with some cheese, which is the next food to be added to your list.

One Serving of Cheese per Day

What cheese are you allowed to eat, and how much?

You may eat all hard-rind cheeses, such as cheddar, Swiss cheese, Gouda and other cheeses from Holland, Tomme de Savoie (a hard French cheese from the Alps), Mimolette, Emmental. Avoid fermented cheese for now, such as blue cheese, Brie, Camembert, or goat cheese. As for how much, you should eat a 1½-ounce (40-gram) serving. I am not usually in favor of weighing food, but since the Consolidation phase will not last too long, this is a good standard serving that satisfies most appetites. Choose whichever meal suits you best, but remember only 1 serving per day.

What about reduced-fat or diet cheeses? Many are of poor quality, so if you cannot find a good one, I would advise against eating food that has lost most of its flavor. If you enjoy soy cheeses, a 1½-ounce portion is acceptable.

Two Servings of "Starchy" Foods per Week

Up until now you have been allowed to eat the reintroduced foods every day. Starchy foods, however, will be reintroduced gradually. After calculating how long your Consolidation phase will last, based on 5 days for every pound lost, divide this phase into two equal halves. In the first half you are allowed 1 serving of starchy foods per week; in the second, 2 servings per week. This approach avoids the risk of your starting to eat sugar-rich foods too suddenly.

Starchy foods refer to potatoes, foods made from flour, such as breads and pasta, as well as cereals such as rice and corn. In the Consolidation phase, in which prudence is the rule, all starches are not of equal value, and I list them for you here in descending order of interest.

- *Pasta* made of durum wheat is the starch best adapted for our particular use; whole grain varieties are also useful. Moreover, everyone likes pasta, and it is rarely associated with dieting, so it is a source of comfort for dieters who have been working so hard to lose weight. Finally, and most important, pasta has a filling and satisfying consistency. Its only drawback is that it is often cooked with butter, oil, or cream, as well as cheese, which then doubles the calorie intake.

So eat pasta, and take a healthy 8-ounce (225-gram) serving cooked (about 2 ounces of uncooked pasta), but avoid oil and opt instead for a nice sauce of fresh tomatoes, onions, and spices, with a light sprinkling of Parmesan cheese. If you are in a hurry, use a jarred sauce made without sugar or canned tomatoes.

- *Couscous, bulgur wheat, and wheat berries* have the same beneficial properties as pasta. Whole wheat couscous is also available.
- *Polenta, quinoa, and millet* are also whole grains, and you may eat the same quantity of them—an 8-ounce (225-gram) serving cooked.
- *Lentils and other legumes like lima beans, kidney beans, white beans, butter beans, chick peas, split peas, dried peas, and dried beans of all colors* also provide excellent nutrition. Unfortunately, they do take time to prepare and have a reputation for causing flatulence. But for those who like them and digest them well, they are an excellent stabilization food and very satisfying. You are allowed an 8-ounce (225-gram) serving cooked. Once again, no oil, but do serve with tomatoes, onions, and spices—a bay leaf works well.
- *Rice and potatoes* are also allowed, but, as you can see, they appear at the bottom of our list and so can only be eaten occasionally. Priority should be given to the foods listed earlier in our list. If possible, it is better to eat brown rice, without butter or oil, as it is assimilated more slowly because of its fiber. Or choose the tastier varieties such as basmati and wild rice. Each serving must not exceed 6 ounces (175 grams) of white rice or 8 ounces (225 grams) of brown rice, cooked.

As for potatoes, prepare them baked in their skin or boiled, and always without any butter or sauce. French fries or, even worse, potato chips are among the few foods that I advise you to forget about totally, not only because they are full of fat and calories, but because they are detrimental to your overall health.

New Meats You Can Add to Your Diet

Up until now you were allowed the lean meats. From now on you can add lamb and roast pork as well as ham, in any quantity, once or twice a week.

- *Leg of lamb* is the leanest part of the animal, but avoid eating the outer slices of the roast. First, the fat surrounding the leg does not come away easily, so the first slices are high in fat and calories. Second, large roasts are usually cooked to a very high surface temperature to ensure that they are properly cooked inside. But this often chars the outside layer, making it potentially carcinogenic. If you like your meat well done, take the second slice.
- *Cooked ham* may now be eaten. You are no longer limited solely to rindless extra-lean ham. You may eat all kinds of ham, but be careful to remove all fat. However, avoid cured hams such as prosciutto, which are not allowed yet.

These food categories are the platform for your transition diet. Remember that this is not at all a permanent diet or a weight loss diet. This is a healthy, balanced diet whose only role is to help you get through a period when your body, worried about losing its reserves, is doing all it can to restore them.

Five days for every pound lost is about the time you need to reassure your body and for it to come to terms with the new weight you are trying to impose on it. Once you get beyond this transition period, you will be free to eat as you want for 6 days out of 7. This prospect should give you the encouragement and patience you need; you know where you are heading and how long it will take.

But that is not all. To conclude this transition diet, I have two more important things to tell you. I will start with the good news.

Two Celebration Meals per Week

During the first half of the Consolidation phase you are allowed 1 celebration meal per week; during the second half you are allowed 2. For example: You have just lost 20 pounds, so your Consolidation phase will last 100 days. The first 50 days, you are allowed 1 serving of starchy foods per week and 1 celebration meal per week. For the remaining 50 days, you can have 2 servings of starchy foods per week and 2 celebration meals per week. I really want to emphasize the word *meal* here because even when I write it out on a prescription, some patients seem to think that it means "all day long."

What is a celebration meal? A celebration meal can be any one of your three meals in the day, but my advice is to choose dinner.

Celebration means party time! At each celebration meal you can eat whatever kind of food you want and especially whatever you have most missed during the weight loss period. There are nevertheless two important conditions: never have second helpings of the same dish, and when you are allowed 2 celebration meals per week, never eat 2 celebration meals in a row. Everything is allowed, but only one of each: 1 starter, 1 main dish, 1 dessert, and 1 glass of wine—all in a reasonable quantity but only once.

Take care to space out your celebration meals to give your body time to recover in between. If you have a celebration meal for lunch on Tuesday, then do not have one for dinner on the same day. Leave at least one meal in between. You might also want to keep celebration meals for evenings and weekends when you are eating out.

For those of you who miss fried chicken, spareribs, baked ziti, or any other dish, now is your chance. For those of you who have been waiting so long to finish your meal with a real dessert such as a piece of chocolate cake or ice cream, well, now you can. For those of you who like good wine or champagne, you can now enjoy them too.

Now without a second thought, you can accept those dinner invitations you have had to refuse, but only once a week during the first half of your Consolidation phase, then twice a week during the second half.

Many of you who have got this far will have become so used to eating in a new way that you will hesitate to let go and enjoy a celebration meal.

You should understand, though, that these meals too have been carefully planned. Moreover, these celebration meals are not simply suggestions, they are instructions you must follow to the letter.

The Dukan Diet is a comprehensive program, and you cannot pick and choose from its different component parts without reducing its effectiveness. Maybe you do not fully understand why the freedom of these two meals is so important. Now, then, is the time to talk to you about pleasure, the other aspect of eating.

Nourishing yourself is not just about taking in enough calories to survive; it is also, and even more important, about enjoying eating as part of that process. It is now time to reintroduce this pleasure, this vital reward that was taken away from you during your weight loss period.

Since we are talking about what tastes good, I will use this opportunity to give you an important piece of advice, essential for any permanent stabilization. So do not take it lightly.

When you eat, and particularly if what you are eating is savory and rich, *think about what you are eating*. Concentrate on what is in your mouth and on each and every sensation this food is giving you. Numerous studies carried out by nutritionists have proved the major role that taste sensations play in making us feel full, triggering the feeling of being full and satisfied.

So eat slowly and *concentrate on what is in your mouth*. Avoid eating while watching television or reading.

Enjoy these wonderful celebration meal moments, without any guilt, and, believe me, they will not cost you a thing.

There are, however, two conditions you must abide by:

1. The first is of utmost importance. This freedom is precisely limited in time, and not sticking to these limits would derail your success. Do not play down the danger. If, for example, you have chosen Tuesday night for your celebration meal, you need to understand that Wednesday's breakfast is when the success of your diet is on the line.

These two celebration freedom meals are there to help you hold on until your body accepts its new weight. They are an integral part of your transition diet. But if you step beyond these limits, you risk compromising everything that you have so patiently worked for.

2. The second condition is common sense. The celebration meal is meant to give you a dose of pleasure, but it is not an invitation to binge. Using this freedom as an excuse to stuff yourself means you have not understood me, and you run the risk of damaging your system. Eating until you are nauseous or drinking until you are drunk will throw you completely off balance. Even if you go back on the straight and narrow the next day, the rhythm will have been broken, and with it your hope of eventual stabilization.

If you want a simple piece of advice, eat what you want, give yourself generous servings, but never take seconds. If you eat your celebration meal at home or at a friend's home, do as you would in a restaurant, where you cannot ask for a second helping.

One Day of Pure Proteins per Week

Here you are with all of the ingredients that make up the Dukan Diet's Consolidation phase. You now know what you have to eat and how long this period, easily calculated, will last until your body accepts the new weight imposed on it.

Nevertheless, one key ingredient, vital for the security of this Stabilization phase, is missing. This diet, with the added variety of two celebration meals a week, cannot on its own guarantee perfect weight control during this highly sensitive period. That is why I have included, by way of security, 1 full day per week of the pure protein diet, which you have already tried and tested.

On this day, you eat only pure protein foods. I will just remind you of the main categories: lean meats, all fish and seafood, poultry without the skin, eggs, nonfat dairy products, and 1½ quarts of water. As before, you can eat as much and as often as you want from these protein categories and in any combination and proportions that suit you.

This pure protein day is both the driving force and the insurance policy for your Consolidation phase. It is the price you need to pay during the Stabilization phase to keep things under control.

Again, this price is not negotiable. Carry out this day to the letter or do not do it at all, but you are the one who will lose out.

If possible, always make your pure protein day a set day—Thursday, for example. This weekly rhythm is one of the guarantees of the rule's effectiveness. If Thursdays are not possible for you because of your job or social schedule, make your pure protein day Wednesday or Friday and stick to it.

If for some reason you cannot keep to your pure protein day on your chosen day one week, do it the previous day or the next day, and the following week go back to your chosen day. But do not slip into the habit of breaking the rhythm this way.

You are not keeping to this rhythm to please me, but to fight against your own tendency to put on the pounds easily. You are the one who will benefit from following this rule, so remember that.

If you are on holiday or traveling, keep it up. You should be able to find plain nonfat yogurt, eggs, and some kind of lean meat (grilled, broiled, or roasted) almost everywhere.

Oat Bran

During the Consolidation phase, you must keep eating 2 tablespoons of oat bran per day. These 2 tablespoons are in addition to the 2 slices of 100 percent whole grain bread. If you have become used to having an oat galette for breakfast, keep the bread to have in the evening with your cheese.

Exercise

During the Consolidation phase, you can lower your walking time from the 30 minutes of the Cruise phase to 25 minutes a day. Obviously, this is the minimum compulsory duration, but if you enjoy it and have the time, then walk for longer. Walking is one of the best activities you can do, for the number of calories it burns up—as you are likely to keep on doing it in the long term—and also for your well-being. It is also the one that results in the greatest secretion of serotonin and endorphins, chemicals found in the brain that contribute to feelings of well-being.

If you are dealing with stress or frustration, if you are suffering from depression or nervous exhaustion, if you have been hurt, if you feel abandoned or lonely, go for a walk. I promise you that you will come back feeling better than when you set out.

Do Not Brush Off the Consolidation Phase

I have kept until the end four pieces of advice to warn you of the dangers of neglecting this most important stage in the Dukan Diet.

The Consolidation Phase Is a Crucial Stage in the Dukan Diet

During this third phase of the Dukan Diet, you will not have the encouragement and excitement of watching your weight go down on the scales. You might therefore start wondering why you have to follow this transition diet in which you are not yet really free but are not losing weight either. You could be tempted to relax your self-control or simply go beyond recommended limits.

Do not do this. If you neglect this consolidation phase, there is one thing you can be absolutely sure of: all those pounds you lost with such effort will most definitely return and return quickly. And if you do not put on a few extra too, you will be getting off lightly.

Putting Weight Back On Leads to a Progressive Resistance to Dieting
Besides the feeling of frustration and defeat produced by putting weight
back on, there is another more serious danger with far-reaching consequences for those who follow diets without consolidating them: resistance to dieting altogether.

Anyone who loses and regains weight several times becomes immune
to dieting. What I mean by this is that after each defeat, it becomes increasingly difficult to lose weight again. The body has a sort of memory
of the diets it has been through and finds better ways of resisting new
attempts to lose weight; each defeat opens the door to another one.

Your Body Retains a Biological Memory of Weight Extremes Moreover,
every time you put on weight and reach a new record number on your
scales, the way your physiology adjusts means that your body will then
always try to reach this maximum weight again.

Losing Weight Is the Same As Feeding Yourself with Fat and Cholesterol
Finally and probably the most serious consequence of going back and
forth from putting on weight to dieting—a consequence of which you
are probably not aware—is that with each weight loss, your body makes
you consume your fat reserves, so when you lose 20 pounds, it is almost
as if you had eaten that amount of fat or butter.

Throughout any weight loss period, a large quantity of cholesterol
and triglycerides circulates in your blood. Each time your heart contracts, this blood, rich in toxic fats, inundates the arteries and coats their
inner walls.

The risks posed by these circulating fats are largely compensated for by
the benefits of weight loss to your physical and psychological well-being.
But be careful not to try and lose weight too often. People who try to
lose weight without success once or twice a year are constantly expos-
ing themselves to high levels of cholesterol. I am not telling you this to
frighten you, but rather to warn you about a very real danger, one of
which both doctors and their patients are little aware.

You have succeeded in losing weight, and now for all the reasons mentioned, you must make the only logical choice, which is to consolidate the new weight you have worked so hard to achieve and then move on, as scheduled, to permanent stabilization.

CONSOLIDATION DIET SUMMARY

How long this transition diet lasts is calculated according to how much weight you have lost, based on 5 days for every pound shed. If you have just lost 40 pounds, you must follow the transition diet for 40 × 5 days—that is, 200 days (6 months and 20 days); if you have lost 20 pounds, you will follow it for 100 days. You can easily calculate the exact amount of time you need before reaching permanent stabilization.

The whole time you are consolidating your weight, you will follow the transition diet as closely as possible. You are allowed the following foods:

- The protein foods from the Attack diet
- The vegetables from the Cruise diet
- 1 serving of fresh fruit per day, except bananas, grapes, and cherries
- 2 slices of 100 percent whole grain bread per day
- 1½ ounces (40 grams) of cheese per day
- 2 servings of starchy foods per week
- Lamb, roast pork, and ham (lean cuts), once or twice a week

Then to crown it all:

- 2 celebration meals per week (you are free to choose any foods, but no bingeing)

But also, absolutely and without question:

- 1 day of pure proteins (the Attack diet) per week, on the same day every week and without fail

HOW TO STABILIZE YOUR WEIGHT ONCE AND FOR ALL

Let's now take stock. The Attack phase gave you an encouraging and lightning kick start, the Cruise phase guided you to your target weight, and now you have just completed your Consolidation phase, based on 5 days for every pound lost.

At this stage you have not only gotten rid of your extra pounds, you have also made it safely through the period during which your new slim body has been trying with all its might to recover those lost pounds.

Now that you have achieved and consolidated your True Weight, your body is no longer extremely defensive. Nevertheless it remains very clever at extracting what it can from whatever you eat and at putting on weight, as it has a biological memory of all those times when you have gained weight in the past. From now on, since the same causes produce the same effects, the likelihood of regaining weight will remain if you do not incorporate into your lifestyle a certain number of habits specifically designed to deal with this risk.

Up until now you have been guided by a whole system of precise instructions, with no room for improvisation. From this moment, instead of sailing along the coastline, you will be out on the open seas, with much more independence than before, but also exposed to a greater risk of storms and, therefore, of shipwreck. So it is important that these new instructions be sufficiently simple, concrete, and painless to become part of your way of life.

To do this, and to break the cycle of putting the lost weight back on as soon as the dieting is finished, the Permanent Stabilization phase offers you, in return for four simple and not-too-frustrating measures, freedom to eat again whatever you want so that you no longer feel excluded at mealtimes.

The first of these measures is simple: all you need do is adopt the basic foods from the Consolidation phase as a safety platform. Eat as much as you want of all the protein foods and vegetables, 1 piece of fruit, 2 slices of 100 percent whole grain bread, 1½ ounces (40 grams) of cheese, 2 portions of starchy foods per week, and 2 celebration meals per week. These foods comprise a healthy, copious, and sufficiently varied range to constitute the basis for your diet. Use this as your point of reference and in particular as your safety backup to which you can return to take shelter if you are regaining weight.

You already know the second measure, protein Thursdays, as it was featured in the Consolidation phase.

The third is quite simply a contract between you and me in which you promise me that you will no longer take any elevators or escalators. In France, we rarely live in buildings with more than five or six floors; if you live on a higher floor, then this rule does not apply to you. You should try to walk up the first 5 flights, and then take the elevator. If this is not practical, take the stairs on every other occasion you can. Our contract also includes your commitment to walk for at least 20 minutes a day, every day.

The final measure is simply a treat: you must stick to 3 tablespoons of oat bran a day for life.

Together these measures seem to me the least disagreeable things you could be asked to do in return for being able to eat normally 6 days out of 7. My professional experience leads me to believe that no sensible person who wants to avoid becoming overweight again could refuse such a deal.

In addition, to crown these measures, the Dukan Diet's permanent stabilization is protected by an additional weapon, less visible, but decisive: everything you have learned about nutrition during the time you spent losing pounds, then consolidating your new weight.

As I created the program and use it every day with my patients, I know that by following the four successive diets, the knowledge acquired about the value of different foods and how to eat becomes instinctive and deeply ingrained, and this can help you stay slim and stable.

With the pure protein diet, you will have discovered the power of these *vital foods*. You now know that these foods represent an extremely effective weapon in the battle to lose weight that you can call upon throughout your life.

Throughout the alternating protein diet, you learned that adding green vegetables slowed down the pace of weight loss, but that these *indispensable foods* did not prevent your pounds from continuing to disappear as long as the vegetables were prepared without any fat.

When going through consolidation, you included in successive steps such *necessary foods* as bread, fruit, cheese, some starchy foods, and even, with your celebration meals, some *pleasurable* and *superfluous foods* without any pangs of guilt. By doing this, day by day, you incorporated a hierarchy of values and learned how to classify foods.

It is this progression from different phases, from *vital* to *superfluous* foods, and the training you have acquired that make this program, combined with our other measures for stabilization, an achievement that may never have been reached before: weight that is lost and lost permanently.

Protein Thursdays

Why Thursdays? At that time in my life when I was still putting together the different pieces of what was to become the Dukan Diet, I sensed the need to add one remaining guideline to this phase in which the lost weight is permanently stabilized, a guideline that would remind people of the battle we had fought together.

In fact, it was one of my patients who gave me the idea. Happy to have lost weight without having suffered as much as she had expected, she was wary of returning to "normal life" and did not want to completely give up the Attack diet that had helped her to "put right" lapses whenever she had any. She came up with this simple and clever idea: using the Attack diet for only 1 day a week! A few weeks later I decided to experiment by formally writing the idea out on my prescriptions: "1 day of the pure proteins diet per week." I observed that this instruction was successfully followed for a certain period of time, then less regularly, and finally, it was forgotten altogether.

So I decided to lay down which day it should be and arbitrarily chose Thursdays. From then on, as if by magic, everything suddenly changed. My patients followed the rule and stuck to it, simply because it was not up to them to choose the day and because nothing is harder for a person with weight problems than to have to choose themselves exactly when they are to be deprived of food. Prescribing a non-negotiable day highlights the importance of this element of the diet. If Thursdays do not work for you, then choose another day of the week, but stick to it.

What Is Special About Protein Thursday and How Is It Different from Other Protein Days?

While you were following the Dukan Diet, you were supported and protected by a whole system of precise instructions that left little room for initiative or error. From now on, however, you have no safety net.

You may now eat normally 6 days out of 7, and these protein Thursdays are the sole remaining barrier keeping you from your tendency to put on weight. You must follow these protein days to the letter, because a single weakness or error will threaten their effectiveness and the solidity of all you have achieved.

On protein Thursdays, so crucial for your permanent stabilization, we must select and use the purest forms of protein, which produce the most powerful results, and restrict or avoid any that contain some fat and carbohydrates.

Protein Thursdays in Practice

On protein Thursdays, you can choose from the following list only:

- *Lean meat.* You already know that lamb is too rich in fat to be counted as pure protein. Only use lean veal or pork, which should be grilled or braised. Roasted veal and pork tenderloin are allowed if well cooked. Veal and pork chops are fattier and can be eaten on other days of the week.

  Beef varies in fat content according to the cut. Apart from fatty cuts for stewing, ribs and rib eye are without doubt the highest in fat and cannot possibly be included in our lean meat category.

  Sirloin and flank steak are probably the leanest cuts of beef. You can even find frozen beef burgers and ground beef with no more than 5 percent fat. You can use all of these without a second thought on Thursdays.

  Be careful with other cuts if you are unsure of their fat content. If in doubt, ask your butcher.

  On protein Thursdays, beef should be well cooked rather than rare. This does not alter the protein content but it does eliminate some of the fat.

  If you can find game, it is an excellent source of pure protein.
- *Fish and seafood.* In the standard pure protein diet I allowed you to eat all kinds of fish, from the leanest to the fattiest. Over time, I have come to accept oily fish such as salmon, sardines, mackerel, and tuna, as they are prized for their immense protective power against heart disease and arteriosclerosis, and their fat content is no higher than some cuts of meat. Nevertheless, this high fat content, acceptable for the rest of the Dukan Diet, is not so for protein Thursdays. If you eat salmon, do not eat more than 8 ounces (225 grams) per

meal if it is fresh, and 6 ounces (175 grams) if it is smoked. White fish is your best ally on Thursdays.

As well as the traditional ways of preparing fish, such as poaching, baking, grilling, or in a pan, another simple way is to eat it raw. Marinate in thin slices, like sashimi, or cubed, as in a tartare, for a few minutes in lemon juice with some salt, black pepper, and herbes de Provence. This makes an unusual, fresh and flavorful starter or main course.

Turbot, red mullet, and skate are the fattiest white fish but are much less so than the leanest meat, so you can eat as much of them as you want.

Crab, shrimp, mussels, oysters, and scallops are even leaner than fish. A seafood dish or platter can save you from embarrassment if you have to accept an invitation to eat out on a Thursday. However, if you are a fan of shellfish and you like it in great quantities, avoid very fatty oysters, usually the large ones. Add lemon to them, but do not drink their juice.

- *Poultry.* With the exception of flat-billed birds such as duck and goose, and when eaten without skin, poultry is one of the best foundations for a protein diet. However, on protein Thursdays, a few words of caution need to temper this freedom.

Chicken can be eaten freely, but avoid the skin and the wings, thighs, and parson's nose (the fleshy protuberance at the tail end of the chicken—actually an oily gland). Save these for the rest of the week.

Other poultry is allowed without any restrictions. Turkey breast is the leanest poultry of all, so eat it freely. Cornish hen and quail add a festive touch to your protein Thursdays. These birds can all be prepared differently. Chicken is best prepared oven roasted or grilled on skewers. On protein Thursdays, go for the skewered kebab version and make sure you remove it from the serving dish right away so that it does not soak up too much juice and extra fat. Turkey and Cornish hen can be roasted in the oven, moistened occasionally with lemon water so as to separate the fat. On protein Thursdays, the best way to do quail is on skewers.

- *Eggs.* Egg white is the richest natural source of protein, much purer than any protein powder you can buy. But this is only one part of the egg, and the yolk, intended for the growing chick, contains many complex fats, including cholesterol. Together the whole egg provides a balanced food you can eat on protein Thursdays.

  However, if you are finding it hard to stabilize your weight, or if your week has been particularly indulgent and you want to get the maximum impact from your protein Thursday, eat fewer eggs; or, alternatively, avoid the yolk and eat as many whites as you want.

  Another solution is to make omelets or scrambled eggs with 1 yolk for 2 whites, and, if you are really hungry, add some powdered nonfat milk. But remember that all these precautions are wasted if you cook your eggs with butter or oil. Get a good-quality nonstick frying pan and put a few drops of water in the bottom before adding your eggs.

- *Nonfat dairy products.* Nonfat milk ricotta, yogurt, and cottage cheese have the advantage of having no fat. But what else is in these products? There is, of course, milk protein, which is used to make protein powder, but we also find in moderate quantities lactose, or milk sugar, which is not welcome here.

  Our two Attack and Cruise weight loss diets proved that the presence of lactose does not lessen the pure protein diet's performance and that nonfat milk products, as your only source of fresh and creamy tastes, can be eaten without limit, or at least without exceeding around 1½ pounds (675 grams) per day. However, for protein Thursdays, these products must be selected more carefully to reduce your lactose intake. Compare your nonfat cottage cheese, ricotta, and yogurts and check that for the same number of calories you are getting more protein and less lactose. On protein Thursdays, if you like dairy products, then go for as little lactose as possible; you can be less fussy the other 6 days of the week.

- *Water.* Here, again, we need to adjust the pure protein diet instructions. There, 1½ quarts of water a day is a good minimum amount to purify a body that is burning up its own fat. On these stabilizing Thursdays, however, you should up this to at least 2 quarts for the day, as this amount will flood the small intestine and reduce its craving for food. Further diluting the food eaten prolongs and slows down its absorption, and another advantage is that digestion is speeded up.

  Thoroughly flushing out the intestines like this, along with the pure proteins, also creates a kind of shock wave that keeps the effects going for the next 2 or 3 days and leaves you with only 3 or 4 days when the energy extracted from your food will be at its highest rate.

- *Salt.* Salt is indispensable. Our body is bathed in blood and lymph whose salt level is close to that of the sea. But salt is an enemy for anyone wanting to keep the pounds off. If too much is absorbed, salt retains water and invades tissues already overloaded with fat.

  On the other hand, a weight loss diet lacking in salt can result in lower blood pressure and can cause tiredness if followed for too long. Because of that, the Dukan Diet dictates only a slight reduction in salt during the first three phases.

  But for protein Thursdays, salt intake is reduced. Restricting salt for 1 day is not enough to lower blood pressure, but it is sufficient to enable the water you drink to pass through your system and clean it out. Purifying tissues is particularly important for women, who because of hormonal influences experience significant water retention at certain times in their menstrual cycle.

  For the same reasons, you should limit mustard on protein Thursdays, but you can use vinegar, pepper, and all other spices to compensate for any lack of flavor.

Do Not Take Elevators or Escalators

Not taking elevators or escalators is an integral part of my stabilization program. As I have said, if you live in a city of skyscrapers, this instruction is not practical and I recognize that 5 flights of stairs is a reasonable limit, but you should still make the effort to take the stairs as often as you possibly can. Anyone, especially someone who has lost weight and knows how much effort this has cost and how much satisfaction it has given them, has to accept this extremely simple condition.

At a time when expensive step machines are sold and gym subscriptions make a hole in many people's pockets, why not think of the stairs as a little exercise you can include for free in your normal daily activities? Here again, you see this advice bandied around in magazines; I make a habit of writing it out at the top on my prescriptions and I have noticed that this is far more effective.

Going up or down the stairs makes the body's largest muscles contract and in a short time uses up a considerable number of calories. Moreover, it gets sedentary city folk to change their heartbeat regularly, which is an excellent way of preventing coronaries.

However, as well as getting you into the habit of burning up calories in the long term, this instruction also has a deeper purpose. It allows you, several times a day, to test your determination to never put weight on again.

At the bottom of the stairs, individuals trying to stabilize their weight are symbolically confronted with a choice that helps them measure their determination. Grabbing hold of the banister and walking up enthusiastically is a simple, practical, and logical choice, a kind of wink from my readers to tell me that they believe in my program, that they are following it, and that it works for them.

Choosing the elevator or escalator with the excuse that you are late or your shopping is too heavy is a sign that you are letting go, and that this is just the beginning. A stabilization program to which you are unwilling to make a modest contribution is doomed to failure. So always firmly opt for the stairs.

Stabilizing Fiber: 3 Tablespoons of Oat Bran Every Day for Life

I have noticed that the patients, readers, and Internet users from my coaching website (www.dukandiet.com) who have achieved the best results and the best stabilization in the long term are those who most regularly eat oat bran, and in particular the oat bran galettes (see page 54), which they make a habit of eating twice a day, 1 in the morning and 1 in the middle of the afternoon.

I think that in addition to making you feel full, just like taking the stairs and pure protein Thursdays, oat bran stands guard over you, making sure that you are still on course, aware of any dangers and equipped to deal with them.

In practice, you now must include 3 tablespoons of oat bran in your daily routine. There is nothing to stop you having a fourth one, though, if one day you feel the need or inclination.

A Small Precaution

Insofar as oat bran slows down the assimilation of nutrients and moves waste through the intestines more quickly, I am often asked if it does the same with vitamins and certain medications. The answer is yes. But there is nothing to fear with a dose of up to 3 tablespoons a day. However, I have noted that some patients can easily exceed this dose, in which case it is best to take a multivitamin supplement and, if you are taking prescription medication, to wait for 1 hour after eating the oat bran to take your pills. I repeat this is only if you are taking more than the 3 tablespoons.

PERMANENT STABILIZATION DIET SUMMARY

1. Go back to eating what you want for 6 days out of 7, while keeping the Consolidation foods as your safety base and platform.

2. Hold on to everything you have learned and the good habits you have acquired while completing the whole program.

3. Enshrine protein Thursdays as the day that protects you for the rest of your life.

4. Live your life as if elevators and escalators did not exist.

5. Take 3 tablespoons of oat bran every day for the rest of your life.

If you neglect any of these five measures, you will put your weight management at risk. If you give them all up, sooner or later you will definitely put back on all the weight you have lost.

SOME EXCEPTIONAL EXTRA MEASURES

Those who are very overweight often have a more difficult time losing excess pounds and in maintaining that weight loss, whether because of emotional, psychological, metabolic, or genetic reasons. If you are very overweight, the suggestions in this section are supplementary weapons that will enhance your chances of success.

However, *these measures are not reserved for the very overweight.* They can serve all who are motivated enough to want to control their weight.

From a Few Extra Pounds to Major Obesity

People with weight problems can be divided into three categories, according to the amount of weight they wish to lose.

- People who put on extra pounds occasionally
- People with a predisposition to obesity
- People with major obesity

Putting on Extra Pounds Occasionally

This category includes anyone who does not have a predisposition to being overweight, whose weight has always been normal and stable, but who has started to put on extra pounds because of a specific, identifiable reason such as a sudden decrease in physical activity.

Putting on extra pounds often happens after a woman gives birth, usually with her first child. Weight gain is even more common if the birth has been difficult, requiring prolonged bed rest, or if the mother has had in vitro fertilization or other fertility treatments.

This kind of weight gain can also happen to anyone who is temporarily immobilized by an accident and eats out of sheer boredom, or to people receiving steroid treatment for a medical condition.

Predisposition to Obesity

Some men and women are predisposed to put on weight. Whether this predisposition is "inherited" or due to overfeeding in early childhood leading to bad eating habits, the results are the same. Such people have a tendency to put on pounds easily and to extract an excessive amount of calories from what they eat.

In roughly 90 percent of cases, however, this predisposition is moderate, and the excessive calorie extraction is manageable.

Some individuals with strong willpower and motivation watch what they eat, lead an active lifestyle, and can stop the pounds piling on, or at least keep them under control. My program offers such men and women real security, freeing them forever from their legitimate anxiety about their weight. But where the Dukan Diet can really help them is to get through those unavoidable critical periods in life when simple willpower is just not enough.

Others who suffer from the same predisposition to put on weight, but who are sedentary or have no self-control when eating, experience a slow but inevitable increase in weight. For them the Dukan Diet is ideal. They extract a high level of calories from their food, but the combination of protein Thursdays and regular consumption of oat bran neutralizes this problem. Their lack of willpower or difficulty in maintaining organized eating patterns is balanced by this small sacrifice one day a week

Major Obesity

Major obesity is a predisposition that often runs in the family, leading to such huge weight gain that the body is deformed.

The energy that such people absorb from what they eat is so great that everyone, doctors included, are confounded. All nutritionists have some such patients who seem to live off thin air, defying the most elementary laws of physics.

I have known patients who have weighed themselves before going to bed and who immediately on waking up and even before urinating had found a way of putting on a little weight; fortunately they are the rare exceptions.

Most often, individuals with a strong predisposition to gain weight are clearly obese. It is here that we encounter people who have already tried most diets, almost always losing weight that they then put back on again. For them, the fourth phase of the program is a good basis for stabilization, but it is unlikely to be sufficient in the most difficult cases. For such people I developed a series of extra measures to shore up their stabilization—measures that are useful for all three categories of people with weight problems.

In line with my philosophy, however, these measures are not based on restricting what you eat. Everything that I have recommended from the beginning in this book remains valid, even for those with a special talent for extracting calories from their food. After a successful diet, eating during stabilization must be spontaneous 6 days out of 7.

The three measures that follow are intended for anyone with a extreme tendency to obesity, but what is good for them may also help those people who, although not obese, already have a "weight history" and are looking for effective control.

First, however, I want to give you some vital information about the physiology of your fat cells—information that will help you better manage your weight on a lifetime basis.

Some Vital Information About Your Fat Cells

Nowadays we know that we are born with a genetically determined supply of adipocytes, yellow cells that make and store fat. Normally the number of these cells is fixed and does not vary. It is interesting to know that although this number is fixed, it does vary for individuals, and those with a greater number of adipocytes have a greater capacity to put on weight.

Genetically, women have more adipocytes than men, as fat plays a more important role in expressing a woman's femininity as well as in reproduction and motherhood. A woman with less than 10 percent of fat reserves stops ovulating to prevent her from starting a pregnancy she will not have the energy to sustain to term.

Once the number of these adipocytes has been determined at birth, it then remains relatively constant, except for certain key moments.

When a woman—or a man—who eats badly or puts on too much weight, the person's adipocytes put on weight too. As the person continues to put on weight, the adipocytes continue to gorge themselves on fat, gradually becoming distended. If the weight gain continues, the adipocytes enlarge until they reach the limit of their elasticity. At this critical moment, any additional weight gain triggers a new and exceptional event, completely changing the future prognosis for weight problems. No longer able to contain any more fat, the adipocyte cell divides into two daughter cells. *This suddenly doubles the body's capacity to make and store fat.*

From this moment on, the tendency to put on weight increases. Quite simply, it becomes easier to put it on and more difficult to take it off. This is because you can always reduce the size of adipocytes, but two daughter cells will never again become a single mother cell.

When the adipocytes divide, what was excess weight gain through behavior becomes metabolic excess weight, and nothing will ever be as simple as it was before.

I am not saying this to make anyone who is seriously overweight feel worried or guilty. I can reassure you that my method *does* give you the means to deal with your resistance.

However, because of the consequences of adipocyte cell division, it is important to pinpoint simply and concretely the moment in your weight history when there is this risk of cell division so that you do not reach it.

Having worked with tens of thousands of patients throughout my career as a physician and nutritionist, I was able to work out statistics that enabled me to pinpoint this moment as being after a body mass index (BMI) of 28 has been reached and is going toward a BMI of 29.

Calculating Your BMI

To determine if you are at risk for adipocyte cell division, you must calculate your BMI, or body mass index.

To make this calculation yourself, you need to divide your weight by your height squared. So, for example, if you weigh 150 pounds (70 kilograms) and are 5 feet 3 inches tall (1.6 meters), the calculation is—using metric, which is easier—$1.6 \times 1.6 = 2.56$; $70 \div 2.56 = 27.34$. (Alternatively, there are also many websites that will calculate your BMI for you.)

This BMI has not yet reached 28 but it is not far off. The main thing is to do all you can to avoid ever reaching this danger point.

When you get near to a BMI of 27, be careful and do not allow yourself to go any further, as your adipocytes are very full. And if you do reach a BMI 28, you must take action: your adipocytes are at saturation point and are likely to divide at any moment, making managing and controlling your weight more complicated.

Exceptional Measure No. 1:
Using the Cold to Control Weight

Here is an unusual way of burning calories: making the body use up calories by keeping itself warm.

Imagine a 182-pound man, 5 feet 9 inches tall, with a semiactive profession. During his normal routine he eats and uses up on average about 2,400 calories a day.

Let's pinpoint exactly how and where he uses these calories:

- *300 calories per day* ensure that his vital organs and functions work: the heart, brain, liver, kidneys, and so forth. Very little energy is used for all this, showing how well our organs are adapted to survive; so we cannot get our bodies to increase energy consumption here.
- *700 calories per day* are needed for motor activity and movement. Plainly we have the means of increasing this activity. For a long time I made the same mistake as everyone else and only recommended more exercise. As time went by, and faced with my daily battle against my patients' weight problems, I realized how vitally important exercise is for losing weight and, even more so, for stabilizing it in the long term.

  I have therefore made walking one of the sacred tenets of my method. Now, I no longer "recommend" walking—I "prescribe" it as I would for any medicine.
- *1,400 calories per day,* the main amount, covers our metabolic requirements, and over half is used to keep our central body temperature at around 98.6 degrees Fahrenheit (37 degrees Celsius), essential for our survival. This then is the area where we can and will increase energy consumption.

To do this we just have to accept the idea that the cold can become a friend and ally of the overweight. Long gone are the days when humans warmed themselves by open fires. We have long since conquered the cold, sparing our bodies the task of keeping us warm by employing a whole range of external protection (central heating, clothes), which nowadays we too often take to extremes. Studies show that the average Westerner is overprotected against the cold, and overweight people, with their layer of fat, even more so. No longer adapted to cope with the cold, when forced to do so our bodies burn up huge amounts of calories just to maintain our vital internal temperature.

The technique I suggest here increases the number of calories you use to keep yourself warm. and consists of a series of simple but highly effective measures that I'll list below. First, though, you need to know that the human body has to maintain its temperature above 95 degrees Fahrenheit (35 degrees Celsius) to sustain life.

Eat Cold Food As Often As Possible

When you put hot food in your mouth, not only do you absorb its calories, you also absorb the heat in the food, which provides heat that helps maintain your body temperature at 98.6 degrees Fahrenheit (37 degrees Celsius). Your body stops burning its own fuel and uses the heat in the food.

On the other hand, when you eat cold food, your body has to heat it up to body temperature before it can be absorbed into your bloodstream. This operation not only burns calories but also has the added advantage of slowing down digestion and assimilation, thereby delaying the return of your appetite.

Obviously, I am not advising you to eat cold food all the time, but whenever you have the choice between a hot or cold dish, choose the cold one.

Enjoy Cold Drinks

Eating cold food is not always pleasurable. However, having a cold, calorie-free drink is a simple habit to adopt, and can be very effective. When you take 2 quarts of water from your fridge its temperature is 39.2 degrees Fahrenheit (4 degrees Celsius). After you have drunk it, you will then eliminate it in your urine at 98.6 degrees Fahrenheit (37 degrees Celsius). To bring the temperature of this water up from 39.2 degrees Fahrenheit (4 degrees Celsius) to 98.6 degrees Fahrenheit (37 degrees Celsius), your body has to burn 60 calories. Once this becomes a habit, you can burn 22,000 calories a year, equivalent to almost 6 pounds and a godsend for anyone who finds stabilization difficult.

Conversely, a cup of very hot tea, even if you use artificial sweetener, nevertheless gives you a dose of heat that adds a few crafty calories that few people know about.

Suck on Ice Cubes

Research shows that ice works even better in burning calories. Using this principle, I suggest that my patients make ice cubes sweetened with aspartame or Splenda and flavored with vanilla or mint extracts, and that they suck 5 or 6 a day—especially during hot weather, as this uses up 60 calories without any effort.

Slim in the Shower

Try this simple experiment: Take a shower holding a plastic thermometer (a glass one might slip out and break). Let the water run until the thermometer reads 77 degrees Fahrenheit (25 degrees Celsius). What could you compare this temperature to? A pleasant dip in the sea in the summer!

If you stay under the shower for 2 minutes, your body has to expend almost 100 calories just to prevent your temperature from going down, the same amount you would use to walk about 2 miles.

This refreshing shower is most effective when the water is applied to the areas of the body where the blood circulating is the warmest: the armpits, groin, neck, and chest, where the large arteries are nearest to the skin's surface, so most heat will be lost. Avoid getting your hair wet or showering your back at this temperature as it serves no purpose and can be unpleasant. If you are one of those people who are just too sensitive to the cold, you can still lose a few calories by showering those parts of your body that can handle cold temperatures: your thighs, legs, and feet.

Avoid Overheated Environments

In winter an indoor temperature of 77 degrees Fahrenheit (25 degrees Celsius) encourages the tendency to put on weight. For anyone wanting to lose weight, lowering the temperature to 72 degrees Fahrenheit (22 degrees Celsius) or lower can make the body burn an extra 100 calories a day, the equivalent of running for 20 minutes.

Do Not Wrap Up So Much

When the cold weather arrives, more often out of habit than necessity you get out all your sweaters and warm underwear. At night, many people put on extra blankets, less out of a real need for warmth than for the pleasure of feeling snug. Make a choice and get rid of at least one of these three protective layers: warm underwear, sweaters, or extra bedcovers. You will burn up 100 calories every day by simply doing this.

Wearing tight or clinging clothes is not recommended. We sweat a little when dressed; this is to refresh the body and to lower body temperature and should be encouraged by wearing clothes as loosely as possible.

By adding up all these ways of burning up energy, we can understand the importance of using the cold to help stabilize difficult weights:

Drinking 2 quarts of water at 50°F (10°C) forces your body to burn	60 calories
Sucking 6 flavored ice cubes	60 calories
A 2-minute shower at 77°F (25°C)	100 calories
Lowering the room temperature 5°F (3°C)	100 calories
Going without thermal underwear, a sweater, or extra blanket	100 calories
Total	**420 calories**

Everyone knows from experience just how much it costs to heat a badly insulated house. Our bodies work on the same principle, so we can make use of this and get our bodies to start using up some of those calories they like to hoard.

Cooling your body can be very useful in a tricky Stabilization phase, when sometimes something very small can make all the difference and turn things round. Modest but regular calorie usage to tackle the cold can be that little extra that guarantees success.

If you doubt me, test the technique on your own, and you will not need any more convincing.

If you have a less extreme predisposition to gaining weight, this technique is not crucial. However, you can make use of it at risky times such as holidays, celebrations, and parties, or you can select a cooling-down day you are comfortable with.

I would also like to add that confronting the cold can be a useful exercise if you feel a weakness in certain areas of your psychological makeup, or if you have a desire to strengthen your willpower in areas where you already feel strong. Facing up to cold temperatures can also help you face up to weaknesses in your eating habits.

To finish, I would say that heat and comfort soften you up, whereas the cold makes you dynamic, encourages muscular activity, and strengthens the working of the thyroid. I have known many depressed people who began to sing once they started taking a colder shower.

Exceptional Measure No. 2: Taking Useful Exercise

Most weight loss theories recommend eating small quantities of food and increasing calorie expenditure by exercising. These recommendations seem logical and rational, but in practice they do not work. According to the American Association of Specialists in Obesity, 12 percent of dieters actually do lose weight, but only 2 percent succeed in keeping it off despite the enormous popularity of sport and exercise in America.

Do Not Practice Sports During a Period of Intense Weight Loss

During the Dukan Diet's Attack phase and for as long as they are losing a lot of weight, I do not recommend that my patients undertake any sport or intense activity—although I do tell them to walk. There are three main reasons for this recommendation:

1. The willpower required for dieting is challenging enough without asking for any extra concentrated effort.

2. A person who loses lots of weight feels more tired than usual and needs rest and sleep to recover. Apart from walking, any extra physical activity is likely to increase tiredness and to sap willpower.

3. Overdoing exercise if you have been inactive to lose weight can quite simply be dangerous.

Three Minimum Extra Activities

Although intense exercise is excluded during weight loss, it does play a major role in the Permanent Stabilization phase once weight has been lost, to prevent the pounds from returning and to firm up slack muscles and skin. I ask you to add the following three simple rules to the basic program. Everyone can use them, even those people who most hate doing exercise.

1. *Do not use elevators or escalators.* I have already described this measure in the Permanent Stabilization phase. There it was intended for anyone wanting to stabilize, but here it is particularly important for seriously overweight people who have managed to reach their goal. They can take their time and stop halfway up to catch their breath; they can do what they like between the first and the last floors, but whatever they do, they have to get there.

   I will remind you that any very overweight person who has lost weight is a much stronger individual than a person of normal weight because carrying around so much extra weight all the time is permanent exercise, virtually a sport in itself. So once such individuals have lost weight, they still have the muscle mass and strength to make short work of the few floors that I recommend walking up.

2. *Be on your feet as often as possible.* Whenever you do not have to be sitting or lying down, consider standing up instead. To

get the most out of this, distribute your weight evenly between each foot. Avoid leaning on one foot because then the weight is supported not by the muscles, which burn extra calories, but by the ligaments, which do not.

Do not overlook this seemingly insignificant advice. Standing up requires the static contraction of your body's largest muscles: the gluteus maximus, the quadriceps, and the hamstrings. If every day you stand upright, balanced on both feet with your hips horizontal, you will burn up enough energy to make standing worthwhile.

3. *Walk with a purpose.* I prescribe a daily dose of 20 minutes of walking in the Attack phase; 30 minutes in the Cruise phase, with 60-minute boosters over 4 days to break through a stagnation plateau. Then back to 25 minutes in the Consolidation phase, finishing with a minimum of 20 minutes a day in the Permanent Stabilization phase.

But for the person who has lost 25, 35, or more pounds, these 20 minutes are not enough. Walking home from work, walking to the shops, walking to see a neighbor—all give your body some purpose again. If you have lost this much weight, you will have to relearn how to use your body, which you once considered, and understandably so, as just another weight to carry around and a burden to your freedom.

Leaving extra pounds behind does not happen by waving a magic wand; it involves reeducating yourself, which takes place in the mind, and you have to want to do it. This requires working on yourself, but it reaps such satisfying results that any concessions are well worth it.

One day a week of pure proteins, 3 tablespoons of oat bran, flirting with the cold, standing up when possible, walking whenever you can, and not taking elevators or escalators—are all minor inconveniences compared with the benefits of liberty, dignity, and feeling normal again.

Exceptional Measure #3:
Three Changes to the Way You Eat

Making these simple behavioral changes can dramatically increase your ability to maintain your weight loss, which psychologically reinforces stabilization.

Eat Slowly and Chew Your Food Thoroughly

A British study showed that a group of women of normal weight chewed for twice as long as the group of obese women, which meant that they felt satisfied sooner and had less need to fill up on starchy foods and sugars in the hours following their meal.

There are two ways of feeling satisfied from food: the mechanical satisfaction that you get from filling your stomach; and the real satiety that comes after the food has been digested and gets into your bloodstream and then to your brain. People who eat very quickly have to rely on filling their stomachs to calm their appetite. This may require enormous quantities of food, which explains why they feel sleepy and bloated after meals.

On the other hand, a person who eats slowly and chews carefully is allowing time to feel satisfied. Such a person starts to feel full halfway through a meal and often turns down dessert.

I realize that it is difficult to totally change this type of firmly rooted behavior. I also know how exasperating it can be if you are a hare to have to eat alongside a tortoise.

Accept the idea that a measure as simple as this can make a real difference. Be aware too that deliberately slowing down the speed at which you swallow is much easier than it seems. The effort involved in deliberately making sure you chew every mouthful slowly only lasts a few days before it becomes automatic and eventually a habit.

On this subject, I have a story about one of my patients. An Indian gentleman who was once obese lost his weight by following the advice of a guru in a New Delhi ashram who said: "At each meal, eat and chew as you would normally, but just when you are about to swallow, push the food back to the front of your mouth and chew it for a second time. In two years you will be back at your normal weight again."

Drink a Lot at Mealtimes

No one knows exactly where this idea started, but people seem to have the notion that if you want to lose weight, you should not drink when you eat. This is completely absurd. Drinking at mealtimes is good for three sound reasons:

1. Water is filling, and when mixed with food it expands the stomach, producing a feeling of fullness and satisfaction. A wet sponge takes up more space than a dry one.
2. Drinking with meals enables the absorption of solid food to be momentarily interrupted. This pause, as the taste buds are rinsed, slows the meal down, allowing the chemicals that send out messages of satisfaction more time to pass through the blood and reach the brain so that you stop feeling hungry.
3. Finally, cold, or even slightly cooled water, lowers the overall temperature of the food in the stomach, which then needs to be warmed up before entering the bloodstream, which takes time and burns up extra calories.

    In practice, to take full advantage of all these reasons for drinking water with meals, it is best to drink it cold. Drink a large glass before your meal, another during the meal, and one last glass before you leave the table.

Never Take Second Helpings of the Same Dish

During the Consolidation phase—the transition between the weight loss period and the Permanent Stabilization phase—the diet opens the door to a number of additional food choices and two celebration meals along with the commonsense recommendation "Never take seconds."

Anyone who wants to lose weight is well advised to follow this one rule, which most naturally thin people do spontaneously. Serve yourself a large portion at the start of the meal, knowing that there will be no seconds. You will eat with a better appetite, and you can take your time. As soon as you feel tempted to ask for more, you are on dangerous ground. Put your plate down and think about the next course.

What could be easier? Drink when you eat, chew properly so that you can concentrate on all the flavors in your mouth, and never take a second helping of the same dish. These rules are simple, and effective when applied at the table, the very spot where your high-risk eating habits, which are in part responsible for your extra pounds in the first place, hold sway.

These instructions, which you can depend on, act like beacons on the road to stabilization. They continually confirm the significance, the scope, and the permanence of this huge challenge, which is to live comfortably and to eat for the rest of your life, 6 days out of 7, just like everybody else.

THE PROGRAM: FROM CHILDHOOD THROUGH TO MENOPAUSE

Especially today, it has become difficult to achieve and maintain a normal weight without some special method.

As I write these lines, in the headquarters and laboratories of the largest food-manufacturing companies there are marketing geniuses, professional psychologists, and experts on the deeper motives of human behavior all working quietly away on snacks of various shapes and colors, with slogans and advertising campaigns that are so sophisticated that resisting their temptation is virtually impossible.

In other laboratories, equally expert researchers and technicians are working away to discover and promote methods and appliances whose innovative features aim to reduce even further the human body's activity and movement in order to present us with products that, according to your point of view, either relieve us from or deprive us of a whole array of practical activities and the calories they would be helping us burn up.

This is all to say that, apart from professional athletes, people living in an elite consumer society have great difficulty in regulating their body weight, yet culturally and socially it has become incorrect to be overweight, both for health reasons and because of the prevailing cultural stereotype that to be attractive you must be thin.

I designed my program so that its basic structure could be easily understood. The only parameters given have been for the length of dieting and the amount of weight to be lost. Now it is time to see how this can evolve and be adapted for different ages and stages in our lives.

The Dukan Diet in Childhood

In just one generation, television, computer games, and the Internet have glued our children to the television and the computer screen as they consume an array of candy and salty, fatty snacks with irresistible flavors promoted by equally irresistible commercials.

The epidemic of North American obesity started in the 1960s and took hold of the youth of that generation. Today those overweight children have become today's fat moms and dads, and the United States has the highest rate of obesity in the world.

Pediatricians in my country have already noted the first signs of this cultural invasion. The rate of childhood obesity in Europe is increasing as children adopt American fast food, pizza, ice cream, sodas, candy bars, popcorn, and sugary breakfast cereals, combined with "computer game immobility."

As far as the overweight child is concerned, we should make a distinction between preventive measures for children from families prone to obesity, who very early on show signs of becoming overweight, and curative measures for those children most at risk from our consumer culture. It is important that parents be both well informed and firm, and never forget that when dealing with overweight children, preventive measures reap the most rewards. Once children become overweight, they will have to deal with weight control problems for the rest of their life.

The Child at Risk for Obesity

Generally the child at risk for obesity has overweight and easygoing parents, is inactive, loves food, has a big appetite, and is chubby from the outset.

There is certainly no question of starting any child on a diet, especially not one as structured as my program. However, help must be given to parents who want to help their child avoid being an overweight adult.

Our advice is clear and simple:

- Absolutely avoid potato chips, processed snacks, and nuts such as peanuts and pistachios.
- Never purchase processed foods for children that are high in sugar and fat.
- Reduce by one-half or by two-thirds the fats (oil, butter, cream) used in sauces and dressings.

With these few pieces of advice, elementary but effective in the long term, the greatest dangers will be avoided. The child's future health, both physical and psychological, is at stake.

An aware and responsible parent will serve as little fast or processed food as possible, and will reserve candy, cake, cookies, and ice cream for birthdays or special occasions. Parents can draw on their inventiveness to reduce the oil in salad dressings and the butter on pasta and bread and in sauces for meat, fish, and poultry dishes. (See the recipes for sauces, mayonnaise, and dressings on pages 176–89.)

The Overweight Child

When dealing with a child under age ten who is becoming overweight, parents should adopt a relaxed approach, aiming to stabilize the child's weight at this point so that the nutritional demands for the child's natural growth will use up the extra pounds. To achieve this end, apply the aforementioned measures regarding snacks, processed foods, and sauces and dressings for three months to correct the balance of fats and sugar in the child's diet.

If the child's weight continues to go up regardless of these measures, use the Consolidation phase in my program, with its 2 celebration meals but without the protein Thursdays, which are too extreme for a child of this age.

If the child is over age 10 and is by constitution overweight, you can now try to gradually reduce these extra pounds. Start with the whole Consolidation phase as before, using the day of proteins to keep on track, but with the addition of vegetables. The aim here is to enable children to lose weight without force or frustration, knowing that they have the great advantage of their growing bodies, which will use up this extra weight for their natural growth.

The Dukan Diet in Adolescence

In normal circumstances, adolescence is the time when boys are least likely to become overweight, as it is a time of rapid growth and lots of activity, when burning up energy neutralizes any weight gain.

However, it is not the same for adolescent girls, who go through a period of hormonal instability reflected in irregular menstrual periods and weight gain concentrated in the thighs, hips, or knees. As their bodies change, girls often become emotionally hypersensitive and obsessed with being thin.

The Adolescent Girl at Risk for Weight Gain

- If a girl simply tends to be a bit chubby during this stage of irregular periods and noticeable premenstrual syndrome, you should consult your doctor, who can estimate the maturity of her bone structure and how much more growth her body is likely to undergo.
- If the girl is still growing, my Consolidation phase is best

suited for this situation and is usually enough to get her weight under control, provided it is followed correctly and includes protein Thursdays.

- If the girl has finished growing, or if she has not lost enough weight following the Consolidation phase, get her to follow the Cruise phase. However, instead of alternating days of pure protein with days of proteins and vegetables, she will have proteins and vegetables every day.

- Should the girl's weight gain get worse, from age 17 she may follow the full adult Cruise phase, using the 1/1 rhythm— that is, pure proteins one day, then proteins + vegetables the next—until she reaches her True Weight, taking her age into account. Her goal must not be some self-selected weight termed as an ideal weight. Not only is this unrealistic, but it will put her at risk for making her body used to a diet that is too restrictive during adolescence.

The Obese Girl in Adolescence

If after age 18, a girl is definitely overweight, has regular periods, and has no eating disorders such as bulimia or compulsive eating, she should follow my program without modification, beginning with 3 to 5 days of the Attack phase, then moving to the Cruise phase, with an alternating rhythm of 1 day of pure proteins followed by 1 day of pure proteins + vegetables.

For adolescent girls, it is even more crucial to consolidate the target weight with the Consolidation phase, then move on to the Permanent Stabilization phase.

The Dukan Diet and Women on the Pill

The new low-dosage contraceptive minipills have considerably reduced the risk of weight gain associated with earlier birth control pills.

Nevertheless, whatever dosage is used, the first months of taking a contraceptive pill are a time when women put on weight, and for anyone who has never had to watch what they eat, it is often difficult to get rid of these pounds. The tendency to gain weight gradually lessens over 3 or 4 months, a short period during which it is wise to take a few precautions.

Preventing Weight Gain

If you have a personal or family predisposition to putting on weight or are using a high-dose contraceptive pill, a simple and effective method of preventing weight gain is to use my Permanent Stabilization phase. If this does not work or does not produce the desired results, follow the complete Consolidation phase with protein Thursdays.

If You Are Already Overweight

- If you are not very overweight, start with the 1/1 version of the Cruise phase—1 day of pure proteins followed by 1 day of pure proteins + vegetables—until you get back down to your normal weight. Then follow the Consolidation phase, 5 days for every pound lost, followed by the Permanent Stabilization phase for at least 4 months so that you do not run the risk of regaining the lost weight right away.
- If you are very overweight, follow the entire program, through all the stages, sticking to protein Thursdays for 1 year.

The Dukan Diet and Pregnancy

The ideal weight gain during pregnancy is between 25 and 35 pounds depending on height, age, and the number of previous pregnancies. Women predisposed to weight gain may put on a lot more during pregnancy. Thanks to the many different features of my program's approach, all possibilities can be easily managed.

During Pregnancy

- *Simple prevention and monitoring.* Prevention is the best strategy for women who have already put on too much weight in previous pregnancies, for women with a history of diabetes or diabetes in their family, and also for those who simply want to take care of their figure. Begin the Consolidation phase, adapted for pregnancy, as soon as possible, and follow it throughout the entire pregnancy, with the following changes:
    - Eat 2 portions of fruit per day instead of 1.
    - Instead of nonfat dairy products, use 1 percent and low-fat (less than 2 percent) milk and milk products.
    - Leave out protein Thursdays.
- *If you were already overweight before becoming pregnant.* To avoid becoming seriously overweight, follow the Consolidation phase, eliminating all starchy foods, and the 2 celebration meals, but keeping protein Thursdays.
- *If you are clearly obese with a high risk of complications for either the fetus or yourself during pregnancy or delivery.* The Cruise phase may be used, especially at the beginning of the pregnancy. Even the Attack phase may be used at this time, but only with the advice and guidance of a doctor. In such exceptional circumstances, the advantages and disadvantages of such strict dieting have to be weighed against each other for mother and baby.

After Delivery

Now comes the classic situation of trying to get back down to your previous weight by losing the "baby weight." However, every woman should know that it is not always easy or even desirable to return to her exact pre-pregnancy weight. Based on my experience in this area, I have calculated how a woman's weight should change depending on her age and number of pregnancies.

For example, compared with a young (20 years) woman's weight, I consider that between the ages of 20 and 50 the average weight increase is about 2 pounds for every 10 years, plus around 4½ pounds for each child. So a woman who weighs 110 pounds at age 20 weighs 120 pounds at age 25 (including the 9 pounds she has gained from two pregnancies). At age 30 she weighs 121 pounds. At age 40 she weighs 123 pounds, and now at age 50 she weighs 125 pounds.

- *If you are breastfeeding.* However much weight you have put on, if you are breastfeeding, it is impossible to follow an overly strict diet that would affect the newborn baby's nutrition.

  I recommend eating as if you were simply managing your weight during a normal pregnancy, following the Consolidation phase, made easier by
  - Having 2 portions of fruit per day instead of 1.
  - Using 1 percent fat milk and milk products instead of nonfat ones.
  - Leaving out protein Thursdays.
- *If you are not breastfeeding.* If you are not breastfeeding, you may start losing weight as soon as you get home from hospital. If your weight gain during pregnancy was normal and a week after the delivery you have between 12 and 16 extra pounds, you can return to your normal weight by following the Cruise phase with a 1/1 alternating rhythm, 1 day of pure proteins followed by 1 day of pure proteins + vegetables. Follow this without interruption until you get back down to your desired weight. Continue on the Consolidation phase of 5 days for every pound lost, and finally the Permanent Stabilization phase and its three measures: protein Thursdays, no elevators or escalators, and 3 tablespoons of oat bran a day for at least 4 months.

  If you still have between 22 and 45 extra pounds a week after giving birth, you will have to follow the entire program with a rapid kick start of 5 days on the pure protein Attack phase, moving to the alternating rhythm of the Cruise phase, then the Consolidation diet, and finally the Permanent Stabilization phase with protein Thursdays, no elevators or escalators, and 3 tablespoons of oat bran a day for at least 1 year, or even longer for women who have not been able to control their weight in the past.

The Dukan Diet and Perimenopause and Menopause

Menopause

Our life expectancy has increased dramatically; currently it's eighty years for women. The average age for menopause is fifty-one, and this change is no longer considered the beginning of the end but the beginning of the second part of life.

Perimenopause and the first six months of confirmed menopause is a time of hormonal change when women most often put on weight. The body gradually burns up fewer calories with the combined effects of age, reduction in muscle mass, and sometimes lower levels of thyroid hormones. At the same time, the ovaries produce irregular amounts of estrogen and progesterone.

The combined effects of these factors causes weight gain that does not respond to the ordinary dietary measures that most women use to control their weight.

If you have reached confirmed menopause, you may tend to put on even more weight.

Vegetable Hormones: A Natural Alternative for Women at Risk of Weight Gain

Much controversy surrounds the risks connected with replacement hormone therapy. To tackle the difficulties sometimes encountered during menopause, including hot flashes and weight gain, a totally vegetable-based treatment is of particular interest to us here in relation to controlling weight gain during this time.

Soybeans and some other food plants contain compounds called isoflavones and phytoestrogens which produce a variety of mild hormonal actions in the body. Although less active than female hormones, it has been clinically proven that they give protection from hot flashes. Furthermore, it seems that regular use of the phytoestrogens, particularly those found in soybeans, provided they are used in sufficient quantity, enables women, particularly those already overweight or likely to become so, to avoid inevitable menopausal weight gain.

However, since phytoestrogens are 1,000 to 2,000 times less powerful than a woman's natural hormones, most doses available in gel or pill form are not high enough to deal with weight risks. According to Japanese research, women in that country do not experience hot flashes and their weight is stable throughout perimenopause and menopause because they regularly eat 7 ounces (200 grams) of tofu daily—7 ounces of tofu provides a daily 100-milligram dose of soy isoflavones, a dose that seems to have the best chance of helping with weight control.

All the authors who have studied the nutritional properties of soy insist that, although its protective action very quickly tackles certain menopausal symptoms, such as hot flashes and aging of the skin, to exploit its preventive effects against breast cancer, osteoporosis, and weight gain it has to be used over a long period of time. Asian women have a surprising immunity to these diseases, which may be due to the fact that they regularly consume a great quantity of soy products.

Preventing Weight Gain

- *Normal menopause.* When you have no history of abnormal weight gain or dieting but simply want to be careful, I would advise you, at the first sign of any perimenopause irregularities, to follow the Permanent Stabilization phase with its pure protein Thursdays, giving up elevators and escalators, and eating 3 tablespoons of oat bran daily. In most cases, this will be enough to prevent normal weight gain. You must keep up this defense for the whole perimenopause phase and continue until the body has fully adapted to menopause.

- *Potentially difficult menopause.* You may face a potentially difficult menopause in respect to weight gain if you have always had difficulty maintaining your normal weight and, alone or with the help of your doctor, have continued your tendency to gain pounds. At the first signs of menopause, you are right to be concerned about additional weight problems.

  If the Stabilization diet is not enough to prevent weight gain, I recommend that you follow the Consolidation phase, which is based on proteins and vegetables, fruit, 2 slices of 100 percent whole grain bread and 1½ ounces of cheese each day, 2 portions of starchy foods per week, and the celebration meals. And, of course, do not forget the driving power of the pure protein Thursdays.

  At certain critical stages of perimenopause, it is vital to follow the Cruise phase, alternating 1 day of proteins with 1 day of proteins + vegetables for as long as there is a threat of weight gain—for example, when your periods become very delayed or virtually absent, or when you are suffering from water retention, bloating, fingers so puffy you cannot remove your rings, and headaches. Normally, this diet is enough to maintain an effective defense.

If You Are Already Overweight

- *A recent weight gain.* If you have taken no precautions and have recently gained weight, but it is not yet threatening, I recommend starting with 3 days of the Attack diet followed by the Cruise diet, alternating 1 day of pure proteins with 1 day of proteins + vegetables. Once you are back to your correct weight, use the protective Consolidation diet and the Permanent Stabilization diet.
- *Overweight for quite a while.* If you already have a tendency to gain weight or have been overweight for a long period of time, I would advise you to follow the Attack diet to the letter, starting 5 days of pure proteins, or even 7 days if you have

put on a significant amount of weight. Then move on to the Cruise diet, the 5/5 version, alternating 5 days of pure proteins with 5 days of proteins + vegetables. You may instead use a 1/1 version if your weight gain is not so great or if you are able to lose it more easily. Once you reach your desired weight, continue with the Consolidation diet for as many days as our rule requires—that is, 5 days for every pound lost. Finally, keep to the Permanent Stabilization diet for the rest of your life.

The Dukan Diet and Giving Up Smoking

When I am asked which is more dangerous to one's health, being overweight or smoking, I say smoking. So what is the best strategy to take against these two dangers?

Many people hesitate, justifiably so, to give up smoking for fear that they will put on weight. There are also people who, having managed to give up smoking, see their weight shoot up in reaction, so they start smoking again in the mistaken belief that by doing so they will lose this weight, only to sacrifice the marvelous benefits of their hard work and compound their problems.

You need to realize that the extra pounds that come from giving up smoking are due to two related factors: the need for oral satisfaction and changes in your metabolism when you give up smoking.

The ex-smoker needs to find other forms of oral satisfaction. From this comes the need to put something in your mouth, the need to nibble between meals on snacks of intense and pleasant flavors that increase your calorie intake.

While the need for new sensations brings extra calories, your metabolism, previously elevated by nicotine, slows down, and fewer calories are burned.

The combination of these sensory and metabolic factors means that ex-smokers can put on an average of 10 and sometimes as many as 20 or 30 pounds.

Weight gained while giving up tobacco will not disappear spontaneously if you start smoking again. So it is vital to hold on to the extraordinary achievement of overcoming dependency on a drug as dangerous as tobacco.

Remember, too, that the risk of putting on weight through giving up smoking is a one-time thing and limited to 6 months, so the effort required to fight any weight gain is also limited in time. Once past this period, your metabolism returns to normal, reactions to oral satisfaction diminish, and weight control becomes much easier.

How a Normal-Weight Smoker Can Avoid Putting On Extra Pounds

Let's look now at a smoker of normal weight who has no personal predisposition or family history of weight gain and has never dieted in the past.

The best strategy for a light smoker who smokes fewer than 10 cigarettes a day or who does not inhale is to follow the Permanent Stabilization diet with its pure protein Thursdays, stairs only, and 3 tablespoons of oat bran a day for 6 months.

For a heavy smoker who goes through over 20 cigarettes a day the Consolidation diet is better and should be followed to the letter in the first 4 months after giving up smoking, followed by the Permanent Stabilization diet for the next 4 months.

How a Smoker with a Predisposition to Weight Gain Can Avoid Putting On Extra Pounds

If you have a predisposition to weight gain or have other risk factors, such as diabetes, respiratory, or heart problems, my advice is that as soon as you give up smoking you should begin the Cruise diet 1/1 version—that is, alternating 1 day of proteins with 1 day of proteins + vegetables for the first full month, which is precisely when the risk of putting on weight is the greatest. Then move on to the Consolidation diet for 5 months, and afterward use the Permanent Stabilization diet for a minimum of 6 months.

Obesity and Quitting Smoking

If you are obese, putting on any extra pounds will aggravate an already dangerous situation. Preexisting obesity shows that weight gain is easy for you and that smoking and nicotine did nothing to keep off the pounds. In giving up smoking, you may therefore face the risk of an explosion in snacking and cravings for oral satisfaction.

Nevertheless, the benefits of giving up smoking at the same time as you embark on losing weight are equal to the difficulty because for the seriously overweight person, giving up smoking combined with weight loss frees the body from the double threat of cardiovascular disease and lung cancer.

This extremely hard and treacherous road necessitates very strong motivation and both medical and psychological support from a doctor, who may prescribe medication to ease the lifestyle transition.

In such cases, I prescribe my program in its strictest version, starting with the pure proteins Attack phase for 5 to 7 days, followed by a Cruise diet in the 1/1 pattern, the Consolidation diet for 5 days for every pound lost, and finally the Permanent Stabilization diet, to be followed for life.

How to Lose Weight If You Have Already Given Up Smoking

If you have completely achieved your goal of giving up smoking but have gained extra weight in doing so, it is important to avoid at any price the temptation to start smoking again.

This situation can be tackled by using the Dukan Diet in its most powerful form: 5 days of the Attack phase, followed by a Cruise phase 1/1 pattern, and the Consolidation phase for 5 days for every pound lost. The Permanent Stabilization diet should then be followed for at least 8 months, or for the rest of your life if you have put on a lot of weight (over 30 pounds) and if you used to smoke more than one pack of cigarettes a day.

BEING ACTIVE

The Essential Catalyst

Dear reader,

If you *really* want to lose weight,

If you *really* want to never again put weight back on, you must *totally* change how you view exercise.

––––––––––––––

This chapter gives you the means to increase twofold the effectiveness and permanence of the results you can achieve with my diet program.

The Limitations of Just Dieting

I do not know how many of the millions of people who have already bought this book went on to follow the diet suggested or how many achieved their True Weight after following it. Nor do I know, and this is most important to me, how many managed to maintain their True Weight. However, I do know two things of which I am certain and which I can guarantee you:

- First, I do not know anyone who has *not* lost weight having followed this diet as it is prescribed. Their results may vary depending on their gender, age, how long they were overweight, hereditary factors, or the number of diets already tried. But anyone who has followed the diet has lost weight.
- I also know that a considerable number of the people who have read and used my method have consolidated and stabilized their weight in the long term—that is, for over three years. I know this because my readers regularly write and tell me.

Nevertheless, I also receive letters and e-mails from people who, having achieved their True Weight, followed the Consolidation phase, and started their Permanent Stabilization phase, managed to keep going for a while but then lost their way and regained some of the weight they had lost. Why? I know about all the reasons for such setbacks as I come across them in my consultations. I have analyzed and categorized them thus:

- Some people are not motivated to start the program. The book is on a shelf, unopened.
- Some people have started the program but stopped because they did not have the motivation or energy required to attain their True Weight.
- Others at certain ages or critical times in their lives have found themselves up against physiological resistance from their hormones, or they have suffered from depression and their medication has had an impact on their weight. With all these difficulties, they are vulnerable to stagnation plateaus, brief or lengthy. When they hit such a plateau without support, they abandon the diet.
- The same goes for people who have tried too many diets without achieving results or stabilization. Diets that are too restrictive, too tiring, too lacking in certain nutrients, too inconsistent, that do not work or are not followed properly are the very diets that lead to repeated weight regain—that is,

bad diets. These diets have made their bodies resistant to losing weight, and they also tend to regain their lost weight more quickly when they abandon their diets. Even on as effective a program as the Dukan Diet, people can become discouraged. We also find people who, despite not overeating, still gain weight easily because of hereditary factors and genes.

- Finally, and this is the biggest group, are people who while losing weight, in whatever phase, encounter personal difficulties: disappointment in love, divorce, overwork, workplace problems, or any one of life's many other painful events. When in emotional distress, very few can resist the urge to reach out for food as a comfort, especially those who eat as a natural defense against stress and lack of pleasure and security, a habit acquired early on in childhood.

It was for these high-risk dieters and anyone coping with life's troubles that I eventually concluded that prescribing my diet on its own was not enough. I therefore opened a second front—exercise—to step up the attack and, with a pincer movement, trap my old enemy.

Before getting to the core of this chapter. I would like to start by reminding you why the Dukan Diet is successful:

1. The effectiveness of proteins.
2. The speed with which the Attack phase creates results.
3. Total freedom regarding quantities, thus avoiding the frustration of feeling racked by hunger.
4. The simplicity of its instructions: 100 foods that can be eaten any time, in any quantity.
5. A strong internal framework: the four phases are structured and signposted, from the strictest to the most flexible, each one with its own purpose, rhythm, and bench marks.
6. The diet teaches you about weight loss while you are losing weight. The order in which foods are introduced records in your body's memory their relative importance, starting off with what is vital (proteins), then essential (vegetables), necessary

(fruits), important (100 percent whole grain bread), useful (starchy foods), rewarding (cheese), and pleasure giving (celebration meals).

7. Two out of the four phases, Consolidation and Permanent Stabilization (the latter lasting for the rest of your life), aim to ensure you not only lose weight but are "cured of being overweight."

8. An approach that through empathy and active support helps you manage your motivation.

9. Lastly, and this is the purpose of this chapter, a final point that is perhaps more crucial than all the others: *exercise*.

The Role of Exercise in Long-Lasting Weight Loss

Exercise is the second general in my army in this fight against weight problems—just as important as dieting.

I have always known that exercise plays a key part in leading a healthy life and keeping weight under control, and I belong to a generation for whom being active was a natural part of life. Being active has always been part of my nature and culture, and because of this I must confess that it took me a while to realize the extent to which being inactive and reluctant to make any effort is a hindrance to rapid, effective, and long-lasting weight loss.

It was a trivial incident that brought this home to me. I was waiting in line at a Spanish travel agency where three employees were dealing with customers at the counter. All had comfortable chairs on casters, which meant they could move about without getting up. Two of them seemed to enjoy propelling themselves around, sometimes fetching files that were several yards away. The third employee always got up and walked to get what he needed. He was slim, whereas the other two, despite their youth, already had a paunch.

From that day, I changed the way I approached the fight against weight problems, realizing how crucial it was to incorporate exercise into my program. Not by giving simple commonsense advice, but by recommending and structuring it with as much force and determination as I did with the Dukan Diet. I told myself that if I, a hardened warrior who had devoted his career to fighting weight problems, had not fully understood the extent to which we are currently neglecting our bodies, I could imagine how much my patients and readers might also have underestimated its importance.

If it is true that we all know in theory that being active burns up calories, it has not been transformed into conviction or action. So I started not just recommending exercise, as I had always done—instead I *prescribed* it, just like medicine.

However, in practice what seems so simple comes up against the problem of its very simplicity—it is as if breathing were being prescribed! For example, when I ask the straightforward question, "Do you exercise?" I get only vague answers: "I walk a bit like anyone else" or "When you've got children you can't help but be active." But when I probe more deeply, a very clear division emerges between two types of exercise: exercise with a purpose, when we have to make an effort and move around to achieve practical goals in our daily lives, and exercise for its own sake, dictated by our wish to remain toned, slim, and healthy. It is this wish that make us feel guilty and take out that gym membership. When you realize that people pay to use step machines instead of walking up the stairs to the gym, you can see the paradox.

How can we believe in the virtues of exercising for a purpose in our daily lives when half of the patents for new inventions aim to reduce pure physical effort and gain time, two ingredients that when combined lead to stress and weight problems?

Moreover, walking is almost as basic as breathing, so it is hard to understand its "therapeutic" value, let alone how it can help us lose weight.

Finally, the concept of exercise is not sophisticated or technical enough for doctors to bother with, and when I speak of doctors, I include myself. For years, I thought that patients had not come to see a doctor with umpteen qualifications and years of experience, a specialist in nutrition, to be given a prescription for walking or exercise. How wrong could I be!

As we have come this far together, I am going to try to get you to come a bit further so that you fully understand the challenge involved in adopting this new concept of being "vitally active": PRESCRIBED EXERCISE (PE). To do this I will pose two simple questions:

1. Does exercise make you lose weight?
2. After losing weight, is exercise vital for stabilizing your weight?

The reply is an overwhelming YES to both questions. Now let's look at the evidence.

Exercise Makes You Lose Weight

If you open and close your eyes, simply fluttering your eyelids makes you burn up energy. Hardly anything, of course, but energy nonetheless that can be measured in millicalories. The same applies if you think or recall something. More so if you think, reflect, and solve a problem. Much more if you lift one arm, and twice as much if you lift both.

By standing up, you immediately increase calorie combustion as the movement forces the body's three biggest muscle groups to contract: the quadriceps, the abdominal, and the buttock (gluteal) muscles. Everything you do uses up calories. So far do you agree with me?

Let's continue. Step outside your front door. Let's imagine that you live on the fourth floor. By not taking the elevator you will use 6 calories walking down to the street. You have forgotten something and are in a rush, so you run back up the stairs, burning off 14 calories, then another 6 walking down again: 26 calories, gone in a trice.

Let's move on. It is lunchtime. You have worked for 4 hours seated in front of your computer. You have been breathing, your heart has been beating, and your blood circulating. Simply keeping your body going uses up 1 calorie per minute. Moreover, during these 4 hours you have carried out your work tasks and moved your arms and legs, another 15 calories gone. Your legs now feel numb, so you want to get up and walk; you go out.

And now, to your great surprise I am going to ask you to walk *for 1 hour*! Oh, I realize this is not easy. And why walk when it is possible not to walk? And apart from anything else, this is an hour out of your work time. Let's imagine that you agree. If you walk without pushing yourself but without dawdling you will use up 300 calories in 1 hour; since opening your front door you have used up around 340 calories.

If you lived in a different world, the world of the primitive hunter-gatherer whose survival was dictated by shortages directly dependent on the natural environment, things would be quite different. In such a world, where you would have to use up energy to hunt and capture your food, walking for pleasure would carry a risk of needlessly drawing on your precious reserves of fat. You can see how incredibly important exercise is to managing our human energy reserves. These reserves are precisely what you are trying to get rid of and what these first humans held on to for their very survival. Here you have put your finger on the crux of why it is so difficult to lose weight and how much exercise will help and how.

Let's come back to you. If you are reading this book it is probably because you are overweight. If this is so, each pound of fat you are carrying on your hips and thighs if you are a pear shape, or on your bust and tummy if you are an an apple shape, each one of these pounds that you hate so much stores approximately 3,500 calories. Scientifically this means that you need only walk 1 hour a day, 4 days a week, for 3 weeks to get rid of 1 pound. Take an example: 300 calories × 12 days = 3,600 calories = a little more than 1 pound of your fat. And without changing what you eat. This hour of walking alone could sort out your weight problems. Too good to be true! I can already hear all the objections coming thick and fast. Who has 1 hour a day, 5 times a week? How can you fit this time into a busy working life?

I agree that we all lead busy lives, so I am going to show you how to fit exercise into your schedule and use its impressive firepower, which is and always has been available to us.

Is being active more unpleasant or difficult than dieting? The answer is NO!

Because the Dukan Diet is so successful, I want to add to it what I consider to be no more and no less than a second engine.

Exercise Helps Us Manage Pleasure and Lack of Pleasure

I am now going to ask you to follow me into unusual territory, into life's inner depths, to the place where your first decisions come into being, the place where your reasons for living and not dying take root. This may all seem very far removed from mundane weight problems; in fact, as you will see, it gets right to the very heart of the matter. Come, follow me, and you will not regret it.

If you are overweight, you probably realize that it was not hunger that made you eat and put on those extra pounds. Nowadays, in the United States and Europe, very few people really go hungry. Today people only put on weight because they eat more than their bodies need to function well; they eat more than they need to satisfy their hunger. The woman who eats too much, at the same time cursing the extra pounds that are the outcome, is not after nutrition. She eats while driven by a need greater than her fear of becoming fat. So what exactly is she looking for? What she is trying to do, and often without even realizing it, is to create pleasure with something tangible to compensate for not getting enough pleasure in her daily life. Or she wants to neutralize some pain, or there is too much stress in her life.

The difficulty is that in order to lose weight you have not only to stop using food to make up for whatever is missing in your life, but to go without, to stop eating what you want, thus creating an absence of pleasure, frustration.

This contradiction explains why it is so difficult to lose weight and so easy to put it back on.

And yet there is a path, seldom if ever used, a narrow ridge between two chasms: on the one side you do nothing and suffer in consequence, and on the other you do the wrong thing and fail. The middle path—the one that enables you to lose weight without regaining it—is the one I call "being cured of being overweight."

Around the fifth week of pregnancy, a cerebral center appears inside the embryo that sends out the first beats of autonomous life and continues doing so until the moment of death. Let us call this neurological center "life's pulsating heart." Because of it, we feel a powerful urge to embrace life, and all our actions focus on protecting life: eating, drinking, sleeping, reproducing, playing, hunting, keeping our bodies working, keeping safe, belonging to a community, and finding our best place in it according to our abilities.

Each living species works in its own particular way to ensure its survival. Everything that makes survival easier generates pleasure, and anything that thwarts survival reaps the opposite. Everything we do, we do either to gain pleasure or to avoid the absence of pleasure. This is why we experience pleasure when our body is dehydrated and we drink, or when our cells have run out of fuel and we eat.

But that is not all. Along with pleasure, another far more vital "food" enters the brain's neurological pathways; leaving pleasure to the pleasure center, the other continues on its journey until it reaches the pulsating heart in the deepest part of the brain that sends out our life force. The role of this secret passenger is to recharge life's pulsating heart with energy to strengthen it and keep it sending out our life force.

Often confused with pleasure, this neurological food is of paramount importance. Strangely enough, as far as I know, this vital substance has no name. I have called it "bene-satisfaction," to combine in a single name the dual notion of *benefit* and *satisfaction*.

Eating is, along with drinking and breathing, what is most necessary for life and is therefore one of the most efficient sources of bene-satisfaction.

You can easily understand how many men and women do not manage to get enough of this precious bene-satisfaction. When we are low on bene-satisfaction, survival's strident sirens start to blast out, forcing us to get some. And then when this still does not happen, we fall into depression.

In our often subconscious, sometimes urgent quest for bene-satisfaction, the easiest way to get it is quite simply to eat: putting something in our mouths, using food to produce contentment, something that up until now we have been confusing with pleasure.

Medical cerebral imaging allows us to visualize the effects of human behavior, and the one that triggers the most intense intracerebral fireworks is eating delicious food. As far as neurological impact and production of pleasure, eating is almost as intense as having an orgasm, but it has the added advantage of lasting longer. The reason why it is so easy to put on weight, then, and so difficult to lose it by restricting what we can eat, is because eating is our chief source of bene-satisfaction.

Let's come back to exercise and how it controls pleasure and bene-satisfaction. For many of us exercise has become a burden, a chore to be avoided. However, for those who want to lose weight, exercise can and must become their principal, most powerful ally and friend. Scientists have found that regular exercise increases the secretion of dopamine and serotonin, both of which increase our feeling of well being.

If people who put on weight overeat knowing full well that doing so will make them overweight, then it is because by overeating, they are seeking to create some bene-satisfaction. This usually happens to men and women particularly prone to comfort eating. For such people, exercise plays a key role in modifying their relation to pleasure and lack of pleasure.

What I am asking you to do is to make an effort to change the way you view exercise. I promise you that you will have no regrets.

The Dukan Diet's Effectiveness Is Greatly Strengthened by Exercise

To gradually reduce the volume or weight of a container you have two alternatives: you fill it with less or you take out more. The same logic applies to losing weight. Either you reduce your intake—you eat less and have fewer rich foods—or you use up more energy by being more active and burning up more calories. Ideally you will combine the two. Following the same diet, the more active you are, the more weight you will lose.

Exercise Reduces the Frustration of Dieting

You must accept that there is an energy conversion principle between food and exercise. The more active you are and the more calories you burn up, the less you need to limit what you eat and the less you suffer.

Exercise Generates Pleasure

Sufficient muscular activity triggers the production of endorphins, a neurochemical that gives us a feeling of exhilaration. To produce these endorphins a certain amount of activity is required, but once you start producing them and enjoying their effects, being overweight will no longer be a long-term problem. One of my patients told me that she had never managed to fall in love with a diet but that she had become completely hooked on exercise, "addicted." I am convinced she will have no trouble maintaining the weight she got down to. One of my mottos (it applies to any activity, action, or behavior but in particular to losing and gaining weight) explains why:

> *Anything you do without pleasure annoys.*
> *Anything you do with suffering destroys.*

Exercise, Unlike Dieting, Enables You to Lose Weight Without Developing Resistance

Here we touch on one of the crucial issues in battling against weight problems. When the body experiences weight, loss it sees as a threat, which it is programmed to defend. How does it do this? It has two options: either by using up less energy, or by raiding its fat reserves. The more diets you try, the more your body learns to resist losing weight. This resistance manifests itself in slower weight loss, and the slower your weight loss becomes, the greater the risk of your losing heart and failing becomes.

This situation gives rise to the greatest danger in a diet: the stagnation plateau, a period when, although still following the diet to the letter, you fail to lose any weight. If there is nothing quite as rewarding and encouraging as seeing the pounds slip away, there is nothing as frustrating as watching your scale fail to deliver the reward you long for. Weight stagnation, when long lasting and undeserved, is responsible for the highest diet failure rates.

However—and this is crucial—although your body can adapt to reduced calorie intake and dieting, *it is not equipped to resist calories being burned through exercise.* You can burn 350 calories by gently jogging for 1 hour a day for months on end, and you will use up the same number of calories on the forty-fifth day as on the first. But if you eat 350 fewer calories a day, within a few weeks your body will have become used to this amount, and you will have to cut out 500 calories if you want to continue losing weight.

Exercise Means You Can Lose Weight and Be Toned

Even if you are overweight, well-maintained muscle tone makes you look firmer and more shapely.

For Long-Term Stabilization, Exercise Is Indispensable

Once your True Weight has been attained, it is time to move on to consolidation and then to permanent stabilization, when eating is more spontaneous and less supervised.

However, we all know that life's ups and downs can throw the best established routines into confusion, especially because at such vulnerable times, we tend to seek comfort in food. Exercising uses up calories, which actually means that you can eat more. For example, a 20-minute walk cancels out a glass of wine or three squares of chocolate.

And really, really important is the large-scale endorphin production that exercise releases in fit individuals. Finding pleasure in being active while burning up the calories is the best way of protecting weight loss.

Exercise Enables You to Break Through a Stagnation Plateau

In my thirty-odd years working as a nutritionist, I have noticed that the number of patients I term "difficult cases" and resistant to dieting is now outstripping the number of straightforward cases. Who are they? They are mostly women over age 40, and they fit into one or more of four categories:

- *Women who have a long history of dieting.*
- *Women with a family history of weight issues.* Mothers who come to consultations with an already overweight child and who themselves have a mother, father, aunts, and uncles who are overweight and very often diabetic.
- *Obese people who are so overweight that their condition is impossible to completely reverse.* Surprisingly, they are not bothered as much by their extra weight as one might think. Often I find them to be less determined to lose weight than patients with only a few pounds to lose.
- *People who lead a confirmed sedentary lifestyle.* Those who experience modern times as all hustle and bustle and with the accumulation of chores and fatigue are "allergic" to any additional effort.

When people in one of these categories decide to try a new diet, I know that they are vulnerable. They embrace the regime wholeheartedly and lose the first pounds quite quickly, especially if very overweight. Then slowly resistance sets in, weight loss slows down, and one day the body resists a little more than on other days and weight loss comes to a halt. The diet is followed just as carefully but the scales refuse to budge. The danger here is that motivation wavers, temptation rears its ugly head again, and small lapses fuel the stagnation.

A large number of women who reach the stagnation plateau give up, try again, and sooner or later abandon their diet altogether. With women, it is extremely important to make sure there is no abnormal water retention, no hormonal imbalance, and no thyroid deficiency, because these conditions can derail the very best diet. If test results prove negative, the diet needs to be stepped up—and certainly not toned down.

Especially in a stagnation plateau, when the risk of giving up is high, the role that exercise plays becomes crucial. A body that has started to resist dieting cuts down its energy consumption and extracts every last calorie from its food intake, blocking weight loss long enough for the diet to fail. But when exercise is added to the equation, resistance gives way, weight drops, spirits rise, belief in the dieting program is reinforced, and the vicious circle becomes a virtuous one.

When one of my patients reaches a stagnation plateau, I prescribe what I call a "blitz operation" over a very brief period of time:

- 4 days of the Attack diet's pure proteins without any deviation
- Restricting salt intake as much as possible
- 2 quarts of water with a low mineral content
- Getting to sleep as early as possible (sleep before midnight is much more beneficial than after)
- Adding a gentle herbal diuretic to eliminate any hidden water retention
- And, above all, *walking for 60 minutes a day for four days*

These six elements make up my antistagnation shock prescription, and very often it is the walking that makes all the difference.

Since I have been prescribing exercise as a medicine with a specific dosage and frequency I have seen that even the most recalcitrant or over-scheduled people, and in particular those most resistant to dieting, are astonished by their results. What is more, they claim that they always knew the importance of exercise but did not truly believe it. Prescribing is vitally important because of this gap between knowing and believing.

I am asking you, therefore, to look upon exercise with different eyes, as a formidable weapon that has not before been properly deployed.

I guarantee that if you follow the Dukan Diet from its Attack phase through to Permanent Stabilization, and my prescribed exercise program, you will achieve your True Weight and you will maintain it, however resistant to dieting you are. Not only will you lose weight, you will be cured of being overweight.

The Prescribed Exercise Program in Daily Practice

Many times, doctors have been happy simply to recite politically correct commonsense advice such as "Try and be a bit more active, find time, and make an effort." Put like this, there is absolutely *no* likelihood of such advice being followed.

There are some countries in which over half the population is overweight. Should we say no to obesity, and do we have the means to say no? My honest belief is that without consciously asking these questions, society is choosing by default to tolerate widespread obesity. Of course you will hear politicians warn us about overeating and sedentary behavior, but not enough is actually being done to put a stop to it.

Since you are reading this book, you know my opinion. I see in exercise the strategic element that, together with my diet, gives you what you need to make a personal choice about your body. If you really want to lose weight permanently, as effectively as possible, and with minimum frustration, you *must* follow my exercise instructions.

The most frequently cited reason for avoiding exercise is lack of time, which is a poor excuse. People put themselves through beauty and body treatments that are infinitely more inconvenient and time consuming than any exercise. Here again, it all comes down to being convinced that exercise and diet together form a coalition that doubles your chances of successfully shedding pounds in the short, medium, and, even more so, the long term.

The Main Player: Walking

After humans stood on their legs and walked, all our activities changed forever.

However, in our stressful and unnatural environment, walking has turned into both a waste of time and a loss of earnings for those who manufacture ways of transporting us. Why walk when we have escalators, elevators, cars, and motorcycles?

Of All Human Activities, Walking Is the Most Natural I have deliberately chosen walking to be my ally in the fight against weight problems as it is part and parcel of our humanity, inscribed in our nature and our genes. Walking is one of the best ways of fighting against the artificiality of our way of life. By walking we do ourselves good, and as we gradually find pleasure in it, we end up needing to walk.

Walking Is the Simplest of All Physical Activities Once we learn how to walk, we walk as naturally as we breathe. Indeed, walking is so simple and automatic that it allows you to do almost anything else at the same time. When you are out walking, you can observe and enjoy your surroundings, think, plan your day, talk to your fellow walker, even make a phone call. Life does not come to a halt when you are out walking.

Walking Is the Least Tiring Exercise and Is Feasible for Almost Everyone You can walk for hours without getting tired. The physical effort is spread widely over areas of bones and muscles. For a serious hike, you need proper walking shoes, but normal shoes, even shoes with a moderate heel, are fine for everyday walking to lose weight. Walking does not make you sweat to excess, and you can walk whenever there is an opportunity, wearing whatever you want. There is no need for any sports gear, showering, or change of clothes.

Walking Exercises the Greatest Number of Muscles at the Same Time It is hard to imagine the muscular complexity of such a simple and spontaneous activity. What is more, the muscles most involved in walking are the body's biggest load bearers—that is, they burn up the most calories. The muscles most involved are

- *The quadriceps.* At the front of the thighs, they are by far the body's biggest muscles. They raise and push forward the thigh and leg.
- *The hamstrings.* These form the back of the thigh and move your leg backward.
- *The buttock muscles.* Very powerful and bulky, their job is to complete the backward movement of the step. When these muscle masses sag, this shows that they are not being used enough for their primary function, which is walking.
- *The stomach muscles.* These contract with each step forward.
- *The calf muscles.* These are smaller, but are among the most heavily used muscles when you take a step.

Secondary muscles that are also involved are

- *The pelvis's stabilizing muscles.* These form a muscular crown around the pelvis and include the external abductors, the internal adductors, the abdominal muscles at the front, and the spinal muscles at the back.
- *The symmetrical tibialis anterior muscles in front of the calf muscles.* These raise the foot up so that it does not flatten or scrape the ground as you take a stride. Walking greatly develops these muscles.
- *The arm and shoulder muscles.* These contribute less than the others, but they can be used a great deal in power walking.

That we use all these muscles, many of them fuel guzzlers, and at the same time, explains why so many calories get burned.

Walking Is the Exercise That Most Helps You Lose Weight This may come as a surprise, but walking burns up as many calories as playing tennis and many other sports. Calorie burning is optimized because it is a constant and uninterrupted activity, whereas in a tennis match half your time is spent with breaks in play and waiting for the ball to return. And unlike tennis or other equipment-dependent sports, walking can be undertaken at a moment's notice to fill in some spare time, anywhere, and at any hour of the day or night.

In Permanent Stabilization, Walking Is the Most Useful Exercise As the only activity that can be accepted as part of your core of new habits, and for all the reasons previously mentioned—it is easy, natural, healthy, and free from danger of injury or cardiovascular risk—walking is the activity that people will most easily agree to undertake regularly.

For Obese People, Walking Is the Only Risk-Free Exercise The heavier you are, the better it is to walk. An obese or even an overweight person is carrying a load. Carrying an extra 30 pounds may be looked upon in its own right as a sport, but only if it is moved around through walking.

Walking Is the Exercise That Best Protects Against Aging Walking for 30 minutes a day, as well as helping us lose and stabilize our weight, can help us live longer and in better physical condition. Walking also enhances our mental health. The activity activates the production of endorphins—the neurotransmitters for pleasure—and serotonin, the "happiness hormone." Serotonin deficiency contributes to the onset of depression.

HOW TO WALK DURING THE DUKAN DIET'S FOUR PHASES

As part of my program, walking is to be combined with the diet based on the special features and purpose of each of its phases.

- In the Attack phase, 20 minutes a day.
- In the Cruise phase, 30 minutes a day. If stagnation lasts longer than 7 days, increase this to 60 minutes a day for four days.
- In the Consolidation phase, 25 minutes a day.
- In the Permanent Stabilization phase, you must absolutely stick to 20 minutes a day.

Walking in the Attack Phase

In the Attack phase, walking is practically the only exercise prescribed capable of maximizing results without producing fatigue and an increased appetite. I prescribe a 20-minute walk per day. Unless you already have particular habits and affinities, any more or less is not recommended.

In general, with 2 days of pure proteins you can expect to lose between 1 pound 12 ounces and 2 pounds 4 ounces, or 2 pounds 11 ounces if you add walking. For seriously overweight people, especially if their hips, knees, and ankles are fragile, I recommend splitting the walking into two 10-minute doses.

Walking in the Cruise Phase

In the Cruise phase, I prescribe a 30-minute dose of walking per day. Walking is particularly crucial in this phase. During the Cruise phase, despite the diet, your body will inevitably slam on the brakes and succeed in slowing down and then putting a stop to your weight loss. When no cause for a plateau can be identified, such as high water retention, thyroid deficiency, hormonal imbalance, or use of medicines that induce weight gain, such as cortisone and antidepressants, it is advisable to increase walking from 30 to 60 minutes a day for 4 days. This can be split into two 30-minute periods.

Walking in the Consolidation Phase

In the Consolidation phase, the aim is to make the transition from dieting to eating spontaneously again and having an adult relationship with food. In the Consolidation phase I prescribe a non-negotiable 25-minute dose of walking per day.

Walking in the Permanent Stabilization Phase

In the Permanent Stabilization phase, the aim is to return to normal life and never put on a pound again. This "never again" dictates a minimum but permanent prescription.

In this phase, which I consider to be the most important *by far*, I prescribe a 20-minute dose of walking per day. It is not much, not much at all, to ensure that you maintain your hard-won results.

The Best Way to Walk

When I say "walk," I don't mean power walking or strolling. I mean brisk walking. Imagine you have to get to the post office before going to work and you have no time to lose. Nothing more, nothing less. You can also enhance your walking by choosing the best time of day and by adding some specific extras.

Walking to Digest

Walking immediately after a meal increases calorie combustion by 30 percent. If within 30 minutes of finishing a meal you get up and walk, not only will you burn up what is required for the walking, but at the same time you will raise the thermal effect of digestion, and also your body heat, which effectively lowers the meal's caloric value. So here you have a way, albeit small, of repairing possible misdemeanors while dieting.

Best Foot Backward

Here I don't mean walking backward, but rather making full use of the moment when one leg is behind, to increase calorie combustion and tone "forgotten" muscles.

Seasoned walkers look straight ahead as they walk, instinctively searching in front of them for a foothold. This is called the forward movement time. The front foot is in the air, and the thigh is following while the other leg passively goes into a backward position. The forward movement time sets the quadriceps to work. The abdominal muscles are also made to work, as is the hamstring connected to the tibia, which with each step lifts up before the foot to stop it from scuffing the ground.

To walk better, you also need to work the muscles controlling the back leg. For example, once the left foot has finished taking the forward step, it returns to the vertical position and passively starts to take up the position of back leg. Here you can take control and turn this into an active time. Instead of letting your foot go back like a pendulum, keep it on the ground. When you do this, you will automatically contract the left buttock muscle and hamstring. Doing this burns twice the calories and makes the back of your body work as hard as the front.

Walking Tall

Beneficial at any age, standing up straight, or "walking tall," is a marvelous way of getting more out of your walking. We are not talking just about an exercise here but about how you go about your whole life.

What exactly do we mean by standing up straight? Quite simply, aligning your head with your chest, elongating your neck, and drawing your shoulders backward and down.

For young people, adopting this posture gives them natural elegance, grace, and style. This is an additional benefit on top of the extra calories consumed by standing up straight, because this position gets an impressive number of different muscles working.

For men and women over age 50, standing up straight and walking with their head held high makes them look younger. How is this so? As a simple experiment, look around you. After wrinkles, graying hair, and a sagging jawline, one of the first signs of aging is stooping forward with a scrunched-up neck. To my mind, stooping ages you far more than being overweight. So lose weight by following the diet and walking tall!

Four Key Exercises for Four Key Areas

Many dieters with a sedentary lifestyle don't know where to begin in choosing an exercise program, so I have chosen four exercises that address two concerns: weight loss in the most muscular areas and intensity of calorie combustion. This is also in response to requests from patients whose weight loss has resulted in flabbiness and excess skin in the four most vulnerable areas: the stomach, the arms, the buttocks, and the thighs.

A Body Losing Weight Has Four Vulnerable Areas

After you lose over 15 pounds, a race develops between the disappearing fat and the skin. In fact, fat disappears quicker than the skin is able to "snap back," and this disparity is even more notable in areas where the skin is very fine and most put to use.

Women complain most commonly about surplus skin and loss of elasticity in four areas. I will first list these problem areas and then go on to prescribe one specific exercise for each area.

- *A wobbly, potbellied stomach.* After weight loss, the skin over the stomach becomes less firm. It eventually regains its former contours, but so slowly that it takes 6 months for it to reach its best tone. After 6 months you cannot hope for any further improvement, but you should not attempt anything radical beforehand.

  As for the stomach's potbellied appearance, this is due to the muscle wall's relaxing. To tone it and have a flat stomach again you have to work the abdominal muscles with traditional abdominal exercises. While there are dozens of these, I have devised my own and suggest only one, as this is enough, but it must be done every day without fail.

- *The back of the arms.* It is mostly women whose arms were heavy before losing weight who complain about them becoming flabby. After weight loss, the arms are not as large, but the skin has not shrunk enough, so the back of the arm hangs down. Here again I use a single exercise.

- *Drooping, sagging buttocks.* Women's buttocks are naturally made up of large load-bearing muscles and a thick cushion. A sedentary woman's buttock muscles show signs of atrophy, and as soon as she sheds pounds, she quickly loses her adipose cushion, leaving her with soft, sagging buttocks. For this very common occurrence I use one complete, single, but satisfactory exercise.

- *Flabby thighs.* Flabby thighs after losing weight are mostly a problem for women who put on weight in the lower body: hips, thighs, and knees. With substantial weight loss, the slimmed thighs are less firm and the skin looser. Again I prescribe a single exercise that can develop the quadriceps and completely tone up the thighs, restoring their curves.

An important note: If you are extremely overweight, doing Exercises #1 and #2 in bed will not offer you enough support. However, both of these exercises can also be performed on the floor, with or without an exercise mat.

1. The Dukan Diet Special: Stomach, Thighs, and Arms

This exercise is my Swiss army knife. I devised it for myself and have been using it for twenty years, and for almost three years I have been prescribing it to my patients.

Apart from walking, if there is only one exercise you ever stick to, I would ask you to choose this one. Why? Because it is simple and can be incorporated effortlessly into your daily routine. You do it in bed, once when you wake up, and again before you go to sleep. It is exceptionally effective and enables you to work a large range of muscle groups—stomach, thighs, and arms.

Position a pillow and a cushion on your bed to make a comfortable inclined plane of about 45°. Lie down with your back on this inclined plane—head down, buttocks raised. Bend your knees and with your arms outstretched, hold your knees, either clasping them from above or on the inside or on the outside—whichever is more comfortable for you. In this half-supine position, raise your chest vertically using only your stomach muscles and *without* any help from your arms. Then lower yourself onto your cushion and pillow support. Try to do this 15 times without using your arms.

Once you have managed this 15 times, start again from scratch, lifting yourself up with your arm muscles now instead of your stomach muscles. Raise your chest to a vertical position, pulling only with your biceps—the large muscles of the front of your upper arms—which are much weaker than your stomach muscles. Try to do this 15 times, which makes 30 times in total for your morning session.

In the evening, when you lie down to sleep, follow the same sequence, bringing the day's total to 60 times so that from day 1 you are building up firmness in your abdominal wall and biceps. This exercise also works your thigh muscles and takes only a minute or so both morning and evening.

Every day try to add 1 more repetition to both the stomach and arm muscles exercises, both morning and evening—that is, a total of 31 in the morning + 31 in the evening on the second day; 32 + 32 on the third day; until you can manage 100 in the morning and another 100 in the evening. By the time you get to this point, these 200 exercises will only take you 3 minutes, which is hardly any time at all.

Thanks to this incredibly effective and efficient exercise, your once flabby stomach will become toned and flat again.

2. The Buttock Muscles Special

I do this exercise every day immediately after the Dukan Diet Special. It is extremely effective: the buttocks, the back of the arms, and the backs of the thighs warm up very quickly, very powerfully, and I feel them getting toned. Moreover, to my mind this exercise is fun, for, as you will see, it has a "trampoline" element.

Start by removing the pillow and cushion. Lie flat on your back with your arms outstretched on the bed. With feet hip-distance apart, place your feet about 2 feet from your buttocks. Your knees are bent, and your thighs are long. In this position, pushing down both on your outstretched arms and also on your feet and the muscles in the back of the thighs, make a bridge shape by raising your buttocks toward the ceiling until your chest and legs are aligned on a perfectly sloping straight line. Once you are aligned, lower yourself quickly, bounce off the mattress and go up again until you form a straight line again. The trampoline effect makes the exercise easier and helps you keep going until you feel warmth and tone creeping into the back of your arms, the backs of your thighs, and your buttocks.

Again, start off doing this exercise 30 times and then another 30 times later when you go to bed. Doing this exercise 60 times a day will not take more than 1½ minutes as you do one repetition after the other. If you cannot manage 30 times, this means your pelvis and backside are very heavy, and that your muscle base in particular is weak or atrophied. If this is so, do not worry. Do a little less, knowing that these muscles quickly adapt and that before long you will manage it. However, try to do a minimum of 10 lifts in the morning and then 10 again in the evening, because your difficulties prove that you really need to do this exercise.

As with the previous exercise, try and add another repetition each day so that eventually you do 100 in the morning and 100 at night. By then your chest and pelvis will look slimmer from the weight loss, and toned and muscular from combining these two exceptional exercises.

3. The Thighs Special

This exercise has a double benefit: It uses up the most calories as it works the body's biggest muscle, the quadriceps, which as its name suggests is made up of four muscle sheaths. It also tackles one of the areas most affected by cellulite. It aims to burn up calories and at the same time fill the empty space where the fat used to be with firm thigh muscle.

Stand, in front of a mirror if possible, placing your feet slightly apart so that you are firm and steady, and support yourself by placing both hands on a table or sink. Slowly crouch down, bending your knees until your buttocks touch your heels. Then straighten up and return to your starting position.

Although difficult, this exercise produces great results. How well it goes depends on your weight, where this weight is concentrated, and how fit you are. If you are very heavy—over 200 pounds—you will have trouble doing it once. If this is so, try the exercise without going the whole way. Do what you can. As the days and weeks pass, and through practice, the time will come when you can complete your first whole exercise. Soon afterward, you will do a second, and then you will be away and achieving the ideal number for someone who is overweight, a sequence of 15, which means you are not far off your True Weight.

If from the very first day you can manage this exercise at least once, you can get up to 15 repetitions in 2 weeks by adding another 1 more each day as long as you feel able, and by not allowing yourself to go into reverse unless it is to let your muscles recover a little by going back to what you did the day before. As soon as you have finished your first sequence of 15, aim for 30, but take your time. Adding another repetition every week suits me fine.

Once you have got to 30, you will have firm, nicely curved thighs, and eight little monster muscles, four per quadriceps, which will spend their time burning up calories day and night. This is because the good news about your muscles is that they continue to burn calories after you have finished exercising. Although at a lower rate than during exercise, calorie combustion carries on continually day and night for 72 hours. This is why it is important to keep going and link the exercises to one another. Ideally you should be active every single day.

4. The Flabby Arms Special

Women's arms provide a good indication of their weight problem history. Most women with cellulite on their thighs also have heavy arms. When these women lose weight, they lose it more easily from their arms than from their thighs, and very often the result is flabby skin. There are not many solutions for this common problem. Creams do not work. Surgery is not advised as it leaves too much scarring. Following is my favorite exercise for the arms. It is comprehensive, simple, and effective, and you will find it is the only one you need.

The advantage of this exercise is that it works two opposing muscles simultaneously—the biceps in the front of the arm and the triceps in the back—so it develops the muscles and tightens the flabby skin.

Stand up straight and hold a 1½-quart bottle of water or an object of similar weight. Start the exercise with your arms by your side, stretching down toward the ground. Then bend the forearm of one arm, bringing the bottle up to touch your shoulder. Stretch your arm and bring it back down to the original vertical position. Then take it farther behind you with your arm stretched back as far as possible until you reach a horizontal position or even farther. The first part of this exercise contracts the biceps; the second part contracts the triceps.

The complete exercise should be done 15 times for each arm. Try and do as many as you can, and if you can keep it up, then go for it, as a muscle only undergoes growth when under maximum pressure. Once you have done this exercise 15 times a day for a week, try to increase each week first to 20 then to 25, so that by the end of the first month you can manage 30 in succession. After that, be guided by how you feel, but already your arms will be firmer and more muscular.

Remember too that skin that has become slack after weight loss needs 6 months to completely finish retracting. After this time, do not expect any spontaneous improvement.

Exercise will help you to lose more weight more quickly. You will look better and feel better, and you will enjoy the feeling of success and satisfaction.

100
NATURAL FOODS
THAT KEEP YOU
SLIM

Eat As Much As You Like

MEAT

Steak: flank, sirloin, London broil
Beef tenderloin, filet mignon
Extra lean kosher beef hot dogs
Lean deli sliced roast beef
Buffalo
Venison
Extra lean ham
Pork tenderloin, pork loin roast
Lean center-cut pork chops
Reduced-fat bacon, soy bacon
Veal chops
Veal scaloppine

POULTRY

    Chicken

    Ostrich steak

    Chicken liver

    Turkey

    Low-fat deli slices of chicken or turkey

    Cornish hen

    Nonfat turkey and chicken sausage

    Wild duck

    Quail

    Rabbit

FISH

    Arctic char

    Catfish

    Cod

    Flounder

    Grouper

    Haddock

    Halibut and smoked halibut

    Herring

    Mackerel

    Mahi-mahi

    Monkfish

    Orange roughy

    Perch

    Red snapper

    Salmon or smoked salmon

    Sardines

    Sea bass

    Shark

    Sole

    Surimi

    Swordfish

Tilapia

Trout

Tuna, fresh or canned in water

SHELLFISH

Clams

Crab

Crawfish, crayfish

Lobster

Mussels

Octopus

Oysters

Scallops

Shrimp

Squid

EGGS

Chicken eggs

NONFAT DAIRY PRODUCTS

Fat-free cottage cheese

Fat-free cream cheese

Fat-free ricotta

Fat-free sour cream

Nonfat milk

Nonfat yogurt, unsweetened or artificially sweetened

PLANT PROTEINS

Tofu

Tempeh

Seitan

Soy foods and veggie burgers (see pages 47–51)

VEGETABLES

Artichoke

Asparagus

Bean sprouts

Beet

Broccoli

Brussels sprouts

Cabbage

Carrots

Cauliflower

Celery

Cucumber

Eggplant

Endive

Fennel

Green beans

Kale

Lettuce, arugula, radicchio

Mushrooms

Okra

Onions, leeks, shallots

Palm hearts

Peppers

Pumpkin

Radishes

Rhubarb

Spaghetti squash

Spinach

Tomato

Turnip

Watercress

Zucchini

AND

Shirataki noodles

Sugar-free gelatin

RECIPES AND
MENUS

If you have already started the pure protein diet, you have probably noticed its surprising mixture of effectiveness and simplicity. One of the best things about the Dukan Diet is this simplicity, which eliminates all ambiguity by focusing on exactly which foods you can eat. But this diet also has its Achilles' heel. Some patients, because they lack time or imagination, limit themselves to a repertoire of steaks, chicken breast, extra-lean deli turkey, hard-boiled eggs, and nonfat yogurt, repeating the same menu day after day.

This solution is of course in line with the diet's creed, which is to allow you to eat freely within the list of permitted foods. However, limiting yourself in this way eventually becomes monotonous and wearisome, wrongly creating the impression that the Dukan Diet lacks variety.

But it does not, so it is absolutely essential, especially for anyone who has a lot of weight to lose, to make an effort to ensure that their meals are not only bearable, but actually appetizing and attractive.

Among my patients, I have seen that some people are more inventive than others and manage to create bold dishes and combinations, as well as innovative recipes that make their diet enjoyable. I started writing down these recipes and giving them to other patients who had less time or creativity, instigating a recipe exchange for anyone about to start the Dukan Diet.

These recipes make use of the list of foods for the pure protein Attack diet and then the list for the Cruise diet, with its protein foods and vegetables. They are only suggestions and in no way prevent inventive readers from coming up with original ideas to make their meals even more varied. The ultimate purpose of this recipe collection is to save time so anyone using them can spend more time on improving the quality and presentation of their dishes and meals.

Sauces, Mayonnaise, and Dressings

The vast majority of sauces require large quantities of oil, butter, or cream, which are the chief enemies of anyone wanting to lose weight. The one exception is tiny, almost negligible amounts of vegetable oil (of your choice) when necessary.

The major problem in following my program, in particular its first two phases, is therefore finding suitable sauces and seasonings to accompany the pure proteins of the Dukan Diet.

You can replace fats with several available alternatives, including the following:

- *Cornstarch.* Cornstarch, a cousin of tapioca, is useful for its thickening and binding properties. Although it is a carbohydrate, you need such a tiny amount—1 teaspoon for ½ cup (125 milliliters) of sauce—that it is allowed. Cornstarch makes sauces, especially béchamel, creamy without adding any fat.

  Before using cornstarch in a sauce, you must thin it with a small amount of cold liquid—water, milk, or stock—before adding it to the hot mixture. It thickens when heated.
- *Low-fat bouillon cubes (beef, chicken, fish, and vegetable).* Low-fat bouillon cubes are very useful for their thickening and binding qualities when replacing oil in salad dressings and also for sauces. When mixed with a bed of chopped, sautéed onions to accompany meat and fish, they add flavor without fat.

Consuming raw or undercooked eggs carries the risk of serious food poisoning with salmonella bacteria. Raw or undercooked eggs should not be eaten by the very young, the very old, pregnant women, or anyone with a compromised immune system.

Some recipes in this book call for raw eggs. Pasteurized eggs, which can be found in many supermarkets, can be substituted for raw eggs in any of these recipes with virtually the same results. If pasteurized eggs are not available, in some recipes liquid pasteurized eggs such as Egg Beaters or Better'n Eggs can be used. Dressing and sauce recipes using liquid pasteurized eggs will have a slightly thinner consistency.

Unless otherwise noted, the following recipes for sauces, mayonnaise, and dressings can be used in the Attack phase of the diet as well as the Cruise, Consolidation, and Permanent Stabilization phases.

Basic Vinaigrette 1

This easy, flavorful vinaigrette uses a tiny amount of oil.

1 tablespoon mustard (Dijon or, even better, French whole-grain
    mustard)
5 tablespoons balsamic vinegar
1 teaspoon vegetable oil
Salt and freshly ground black pepper to taste
Optional:
1 large garlic clove
7 or 8 basil leaves

Take a clean, empty jar and add the mustard, balsamic vinegar, vegetable oil, salt, and freshly ground black pepper. If you like garlic, add a large clove to marinate in the bottom of the jar, together with 7 or 8 basil leaves. Cover the jar and shake well to blend.

Variation:

If you do not like balsamic vinegar, you can select another one. Just use a little less: 4 tablespoons for wine, sherry, or raspberry vinegar; 3 tablespoons for champagne vinegar.

Basic Vinaigrette 2

This vinaigrette is a basic dressing that you can use in the Cruise phase to make it easy to enjoy salads and raw foods. You can adapt it to suit your taste by using different types of vinegar and your choice of herbs or other additional seasonings.

MAKES ABOUT ¼ CUP
Preparation time: 5 minutes

1 teaspoon vegetable oil
1 tablespoon mineral water
2 tablespoons sherry, raspberry, *or* balsamic vinegar
1 tablespoon Dijon mustard
Salt and pepper to taste

Place all ingredients in a bowl and mix together until well blended.

Note: For variety, add herbs, soy sauce, Tabasco, or Worcestershire sauce to taste.

Classic Mayonnaise

MAKES ABOUT ½ CUP
Preparation time: 5 minutes

1 raw egg yolk *or* 1 pasteurized egg yolk *or* 1 tablespoon liquid
    pasteurized egg
Salt and pepper to taste
1 teaspoon vinegar
1 teaspoon vegetable oil
½ teaspoon Dijon mustard

1. Place egg in a mixing bowl with salt, pepper, and vinegar.
2. Slowly stir until well combined.
3. While stirring, add vegetable oil one drop at a time.
4. When mixture begins to thicken, add mustard and stir until thoroughly combined.

5. Taste and make adjustments by adding salt and pepper for flavor and more mustard for a thicker consistency.

   Mayonnaise will keep refrigerated in a covered container for 2 to 3 days.

Note: Using liquid pasteurized eggs will result in a slightly thinner consistency.

Green Mayonnaise

Green Mayonnaise can be used in all of the phases, but refrain from eating it if you are experiencing a stagnation in your weight loss.

MAKES ABOUT ½ CUP

Prepare Classic Mayonnaise recipe and add 1 tablespoon of chopped fresh parsley or chives or 1 teaspoon crushed dried parsley or chives. Mayonnaise will keep refrigerated in a covered container for 2 to 3 days.

Oil-Free Mayonnaise

MAKES ABOUT ½ CUP

Preparation time: 5 minutes, plus 12 minutes for the hard-boiled egg

> 1 hard-boiled egg
> ¼ cup fat-free cottage cheese* or fat-free sour cream
> ½ teaspoon Dijon mustard
> Salt and pepper to taste

1. Thoroughly crush the yolk of the hard-boiled egg with a fork.
2. Add the cottage cheese or sour cream.
3. Add mustard, salt and pepper, and other spices if desired.

   Mayonnaise will keep refrigerated in a covered container for 2 to 3 days.

*For a smoother consistency, whir the cottage cheese in a blender before using.

Dukan Herb Mayonnaise

This mayonnaise can be used in all of the phases, but refrain from eating it if you are experiencing a stagnation in your weight loss.

MAKES ABOUT ½ CUP
Preparation time: 10 minutes

1 raw egg yolk *or* 1 pasteurized egg yolk *or* 1 tablespoon liquid
    pasteurized egg
1 tablespoon Dijon mustard
Salt and pepper to taste
1 tablespoon chopped fresh parsley or chives, *or* 1 teaspoon
    dried parsley or chives
3 tablespoons fat-free sour cream *or* fat-free plain Greek-style
    yogurt

1. Put the egg in a mixing bowl and combine with the mustard.
2. Season with salt and pepper. Add the parsley or chives.
3. Gradually mix in the sour cream or yogurt, stirring continuously.

Mayonnaise will keep refrigerated in a covered container for 2 to 3 days.

Note: Using liquid pasteurized eggs will result in a slightly thinner consistency.

Yogurt Dressing

This dressing, made with nonfat yogurt, makes an easy savory sauce.

6 to 8 ounces nonfat plain yogurt
1 tablespoon mustard (Dijon, if possible)
Dash of vinegar
Salt, pepper, and herbs to taste

Beat the yogurt and mustard together until it has the consistency of mayonnaise. Add the vinegar, salt, pepper, and herbs.

Diet Béarnaise Sauce

A classic French sauce, traditionally served with steak.

MAKES ABOUT ½ CUP

Preparation time: 10 minutes

2 teaspoons white vinegar

1 small shallot, chopped

¼ teaspoon chopped fresh or dried tarragon, to taste

2 raw egg yolks *or* 2 pasteurized egg yolks

1. Heat the vinegar in a double boiler.
2. Add the chopped shallot and tarragon.
3. Cook slowly over low heat. Do not boil.
4. Let the vinegar mixture cool down and then pour it over the egg yolks, beating well until it thickens. Serve immediately.

Note: This recipe will not work with liquid pasteurized eggs.

Ravigote Sauce

Serve this classic sauce with fish, hard-boiled eggs, meat, or vegetables.

MAKES ABOUT 2 CUPS

Preparation time: 10 minutes, plus 12 minutes for the hard-boiled egg

1 raw egg *or* 1 pasteurized egg *or* 3 tablespoons liquid
   pasteurized eggs

3 medium-size sour, half-sour *or* French cornichon pickles,
   chopped into small cubes*

1 small onion, chopped

2 tablespoons each chopped fresh chives, parsley, and tarragon *or*
   2 teaspoons each dried crushed chives, parsley, and tarragon

1½ cups fat-free plain yogurt

½ teaspoon Dijon mustard

¼ teaspoon salt

*Use only no-sugar-added pickles.

1. In a glass bowl, mix together the egg, pickles, onion, and herbs.
2. Add the yogurt, mustard, and salt.

This sauce will keep refrigerated in a covered container for 2 to 3 days.

White Sauce

Serve this sauce over white fish or vegetables. It can be used in any phase of the diet.

MAKES ABOUT 1 CUP
Preparation time: 10 minutes

2 raw egg yolks *or* 2 pasteurized egg yolks
½ cup nonfat milk
Salt and pepper to taste
¾ cup fat-free plain yogurt

1. Beat the egg yolks in a bowl.
2. In a double boiler, heat the milk until it is slightly warm, then add salt and pepper to taste.
3. Pour a small amount of milk over the egg yolks and mix thoroughly.
4. Incorporate the egg-and-milk mixture into the double boiler and beat until thoroughly incorporated.
5. Add the yogurt and mix thoroughly. Serve immediately.

When serving with fish, add a chopped small sour or half-sour pickle, or a French cornichon.

Note: This recipe will not work with liquid pasteurized eggs.

Tomato Purée

Serve this sauce with fish or vegetables.

MAKES ABOUT 2 CUPS
Preparation time: 25 minutes

½ cup finely chopped onions

6 to 8 fresh tomatoes, peeled, with seeds removed *or* a
  14.5-ounce can peeled tomatoes, chopped

Salt and pepper to taste

½ teaspoon chopped fresh mint *or* a large pinch crushed dried
  mint

½ teaspoon chopped fresh basil *or* a large pinch crushed dried
  basil

½ teaspoon chopped fresh tarragon *or* a large pinch crushed
  dried tarragon

1. Place the chopped onions and the fresh or canned tomatoes into a nonstick saucepan.
2. Add salt and pepper to taste.
3. Cover and let simmer over low heat for 20 minutes.
4. Let tomato mixture cool, and add the mint, basil, and tarragon.

This sauce will keep refrigerated in a covered container for 2 to 3 days.

Fresh Herb Sauce

Serve this sauce with fish or meat.

MAKES ABOUT 1½ CUPS
Preparation time: 15 minutes

½ cup low-sodium broth—chicken, beef, or vegetable
1 teaspoon cornstarch
1 cup fat-free sour cream *or* fat-free plain yogurt
1 tablespoon fresh herbs of your choice, such as watercress,
    parsley, tarragon, chives, celery leaves, mint, or small
    shallots
Salt and pepper to taste

1. Pour the broth into a bowl and slowly add the cornstarch while mixing continuously.
2. Place the mixture in a saucepan over low heat and stir until it thickens.
3. Take the saucepan off the heat and mix in the sour cream or yogurt, herbs, salt, and pepper. Serve immediately.

Hunter's Sauce

Serve this sauce with meat or fish.

MAKES ABOUT ½ CUP
Preparation time: 25 minutes

2 chopped shallots
3 tablespoons vinegar
2 tablespoons water
1 egg yolk *or* 1 pasteurized egg yolk *or* 1 tablespoon liquid
  pasteurized egg
2 tablespoons fat-free sour cream *or* fat-free plain yogurt
1 sprig fresh tarragon, chopped *or* a pinch of dried tarragon,
  crushed
Salt and pepper to taste

1. In a saucepan, mix the chopped shallots in the vinegar and water.
2. Cover and cook for about 10 minutes.
3. Uncover and continue cooking until the sauce thickens, about 5 more minutes.
4. In a bowl, beat the egg.
5. Remove the saucepan from the heat and add the beaten egg and the yogurt or sour cream.
6. Add the chopped tarragon to the mixture.
7. Season with salt and pepper to taste.
8. Reheat in a double boiler to thicken further. Serve immediately.

Hollandaise Sauce

Serve this sauce with white fish, asparagus, green beans, or spinach.

MAKES ABOUT ½ CUP
Preparation time: 15 minutes

¼ cup nonfat milk

2 egg yolks *or* 2 pasteurized egg yolks

1 teaspoon Dijon mustard

2 tablespoons fresh lemon juice

1. In a saucepan, warm the milk over a low flame for 2 to 3 minutes. Remove from heat.
2. Combine the egg yolks, mustard, and lemon juice in a double boiler over hot, but not boiling, water.
3. Let mixture heat for a few minutes over low heat, stirring constantly until it thickens.
4. While stirring, slowly add the warm milk.
5. Continue to cook and stir until the mixture thickens. Keep warm until serving.

Note: This recipe will not work with liquid pasteurized eggs.

Béchamel Sauce

You can top cooked vegetables, such as broccoli, with this sauce and place them under the broiler until all is bubbly and browned.

MAKES ABOUT 1 CUP
Preparation time: 10 minutes

1 cup nonfat milk

1 tablespoon cornstarch

1 low-sodium beef bouillon cube

Salt, pepper, and nutmeg to taste

1. In a saucepan, mix together the milk and the cornstarch and add the beef bouillon cube.
2. Cook for a few minutes over low heat until thick.
3. Add salt, pepper, and nutmeg to taste. Serve immediately.

Horseradish Sauce

Serve this sauce with fish, pork, or poultry.

MAKES ABOUT 1 CUP
Preparation time: 10 minutes

1 cup fat-free sour cream *or* fat-free plain Greek-style yogurt
1 tablespoon prepared white horseradish
Salt and pepper to taste

In a bowl, mix the sour cream or yogurt with the horseradish, salt, and pepper until a fine, light mixture is obtained. This sauce will keep refrigerated in a covered container for 2 to 3 days.

Divine Sauce

Serve this sauce hot or warm with cooked fish.

MAKES ABOUT 1 CUP

Preparation time: 10 minutes

2 egg yolks *or* 2 pasteurized egg yolks *or* 2 tablespoons liquid
  pasteurized eggs

1 tablespoon Dijon mustard

¾ cup fat-free sour cream *or* fat-free plain yogurt

1 teaspoon cornstarch

Salt and pepper to taste

⅛ teaspoon fresh chopped herbs such as dill, parsley, or
  tarragon, *or* a small pinch crushed dried herbs such as dill,
  parsley, or tarragon

1 teaspoon fresh lemon juice

1. In a saucepan, mix together the egg, mustard, sour cream or
   yogurt, cornstarch, salt, and pepper.
2. Gently bring to a boil.
3. Remove from the heat and add the herbs and lemon juice.

Papa-U Barbecue Sauce

Serve this sauce hot with meat. It may be used in the Cruise, Consolidation, and Permanent Stabilization phases of the diet.

MAKES 10 SERVINGS

Preparation time: 15 minutes

Cooking time: 50 minutes

1 small onion, minced

1 clove garlic, minced

6-ounce can tomato paste

12-ounce can Diet Dr Pepper

¼ cup sugar-free ketchup*

3 teaspoons yellow mustard

1 tablespoon Worcestershire sauce

1 pinch ground cloves

1 teaspoon liquid smoke (or smoked paprika)

½ cup water

¼ teaspoon ground cayenne pepper

3 tablespoons cider vinegar

1. Cook the onion in 2 tablespoons of water over medium heat in a 2-quart pan until soft, 3 to 5 minutes.
2. Add garlic and stir for about 30 seconds.
3. Add the remaining ingredients. Stir well.
4. Simmer on low heat for 45 minutes.

Sauce will keep refrigerated in a covered container for 2 to 3 days.

*If you don't find sugar-free ketchup, use a reduced-sugar brand.

Recipes for the Pure Protein Attack Phase

———————— *Meat Recipes* ————————

Roast Beef

MAKES 6 TO 8 SERVINGS
Preparation time: 5 minutes
Cooking time: 35 to 45 minutes

2½ to 3 pounds beef sirloin tip center roast *or* tenderloin roast
Salt and pepper to taste

1. Preheat oven to 500°F for 10 minutes.
2. Roast the beef uncovered in an ovenproof pan for 15 minutes.
3. Reduce the oven temperature to 325°F. Continue to roast for an additional 20 to 30 minutes, or until a thermometer inserted into the thickest part of the beef registers 170°F.
4. Transfer the roast to a cutting board and let it stand uncovered for 15 minutes.
5. Salt and pepper the roast to taste, then carve and serve.

Cold Beef Leftovers

Serve cold beef leftovers with any of the appropriate sauces in the "Sauces, Mayonnaise, and Dressings" section (pages 176–89).

Beef Skewers

MAKES 4 SERVINGS

Preparation time: 15 minutes, plus 2 to 4 hours for marinating

Cooking time: 15 to 25 minutes

¼ cup low-sodium soy sauce

2 tablespoons Dijon mustard

1 tablespoon cider vinegar

⅛ teaspoon fresh thyme *or* pinch of dried thyme

1 bay leaf

¼ cup fresh lemon juice

1 pound 5 ounces beef top round steaks, cut up into large chunks

4 skewers; if using wood skewers, soak them for 15 minutes in
water first to prevent burning

Onion slices, for flavoring

1. Mix the soy sauce, mustard, vinegar, herbs, and lemon juice
   together. Marinate the beef in the mixture for 2 to 4 hours in
   the refrigerator, turning at least once.
2. Discard the marinade. Place the beef on the skewers.
   Add onion slices if desired for flavor, but during the pure protein phase, discard them after grilling.
3. Grill or broil on medium until done to your liking.

*Note: During the Cruise phase, add tomatoes, mushrooms, bell peppers, and
onions to the skewer. Serve with the steak.*

Barbecue Steak

MAKES 4 SERVINGS

Preparation time: 15 minutes

Cooking time: 25 to 40 minutes

1 pound 5 ounces top loin *or* T-bone steaks, about ¾ to 1 inch thick

Fresh coarsely ground pepper

¾ cup fat-free plain yogurt

1. Cook the steak on the barbecue or under the broiler until done to your liking, or until a thermometer inserted into the thickest part of the beef registers 170°F.
2. After cooking, cover the steak with coarse ground pepper.
3. In a saucepan, gently warm half of the yogurt and add additional pepper.
4. While the steak is still hot, pour half the mixture onto it and then put the steak back on the barbecue for a few minutes.
5. When serving, pour the remaining yogurt over the steak.

Note: During the Cruise phase, grill and serve onions, peppers, and tomatoes with the steak.

Beef Stew

MAKES 4 SERVINGS

Preparation time: 5 minutes

Cooking time: 1 hour 15 minutes

1½ pounds boneless beef chuck stew meat, cubed

6 cups water

1 tablespoon fresh thyme leaves *or* 1 teaspoon dried thyme

1 bay leaf

½ cup low-sodium beef broth

1 onion

Salt and pepper

1. In a large pot, add beef, water, thyme, bay leaf, broth, onion, salt, and pepper.
2. Cook for 1 hour and 15 minutes on medium heat.
3. Let beef cool until lukewarm and serve with Ravigote Sauce (page 181) and pickles.

Note: During the Cruise phase, add a leek to the bouillon. You can serve the beef with Tomato Purée (page 183) if you are in the Attack phase.

Vietnamese Beef

MAKES 2 SERVINGS

Preparation time: 20 minutes, plus 30 minutes for marinating

Cooking time: 10 minutes

10 ounces beef sirloin steak
1 tablespoon peeled fresh ginger, crushed
2 tablespoons soy sauce
1 tablespoon oyster sauce
Black pepper
⅛ teaspoon vegetable oil
4 garlic cloves, crushed
A few fresh cilantro leaves

1. Cut the meat into ½-inch cubes.
2. In a small bowl, mix together the soy sauce, oyster sauce, ginger, and pepper. Put the meat into a dish and pour the soy sauce mixture over it.
3. Cover the meat and marinate in the refrigerator for at least 30 minutes.
4. To cook, heat a heavy-bottomed skillet over medium heat, place vegetable oil in the skillet, and add the crushed garlic.
5. Remove the meat from the marinade and drain. Discard the marinade.

6. Once the garlic has started to brown, about 3 minutes, add the meat, and cook over a very high heat, mixing rapidly for 10 to 15 seconds. The meat should be served on the rare side, so do not overcook.

7. Garnish with cilantro leaves.

Pork Medallions

MAKES 4 SERVINGS

Preparation time: 15 minutes

Cooking time: 15 minutes

1½ pounds pork tenderloin

Salt and pepper

1 small onion, sliced, for flavor only; discard after cooking

1 clove garlic, sliced

2 tablespoons low-sodium, low-fat beef broth

1 fresh lemon

1. Preheat oven to 375°F. Place pork between two sheets of plastic wrap and pound with a meat mallet or small skillet until ⅛ inch in thickness.

2. Cut the pork into 8 equal pieces and sprinkle with salt and pepper.

3. Cover the bottom of a nonstick frying pan with the chopped onion and sliced garlic.

4. Sprinkle the broth over the onions and garlic.

5. Cook over medium heat until the onions and garlic turn a caramel color.

6. Put the medallions of pork on top of the bed of onions and garlic and cook in the oven for 10 minutes, turning after 5 minutes.

7. Remove the onions and garlic from the pan, and in the Attack diet phase, discard after cooking.

8. Leaving the remaining juices in the pan, return the pork to the pan, turn the oven up to Broil, and broil the meat for an additional 5 minutes.

9. Serve with fresh lemon cut into quarters.

———————— *Poultry Recipes* ————————

Roast Chicken with Tarragon and Lemon

MAKES 6 SERVINGS

Preparation time: 25 minutes

Cooking time: 1 hour 40 minutes

A 2½- to 3-pound whole chicken

1 fresh lemon, cut in half

1 clove garlic, diced

Salt and pepper

2 tablespoons chopped fresh tarragon *or* 2 teaspoons dried
   tarragon

1 medium onion, chopped

1. Preheat oven to 425°F.
2. Clean, rinse, and pat the chicken dry with paper towels.
3. Squeeze one half of the lemon over the outside of the chicken. Then rub the chicken with the garlic, salt, and pepper.
4. Place the tarragon, onion, and the other half of the lemon inside the chicken. Place the chicken on an ovenproof pan and cover it with foil.
5. Bake the chicken in the oven for 1 hour 30 minutes, or until a thermometer inserted into the middle of the chicken registers 170°, or until juices run clear when a knife is pierced into the thickest part of the thigh.
6. Take the foil off and let the top brown for the last 10 minutes.

Note: Avoid eating the skin and the tips of the wings. You can replace the tarragon with rosemary in this recipe.

Chicken with Mustard

MAKES 4 SERVINGS

Preparation time: 15 minutes

Cooking time: 45 to 60 minutes

8 skinless, bone-in chicken thighs

½ cup Dijon mustard

1 tablespoon fresh thyme *or* 1 teaspoon dried thyme

¾ cup fat-free plain yogurt *or* fat-free sour cream

Salt and pepper to taste

1. Preheat oven to 400°F.
2. Cover a rimmed sheet tray with foil.
3. In a bowl, toss together the chicken, mustard, and thyme until the chicken is thoroughly coated.
4. Arrange the chicken in a single layer on the foil-covered sheet pan.
5. Lay a sheet of foil over the chicken and fold over the edges tightly so that no steam can escape. Depending on the size of the baking sheet, you may need more than one piece of foil.
6. Put the chicken in the oven and cook for 45 minutes to 1 hour, or until a thermometer inserted into the thickest part of the chicken thigh registers 170°.
7. Blend the yogurt or sour cream with salt and pepper to make a sauce.
8. When the chicken is done, remove the foil. Pour the sauce over the chicken thighs, stirring to dissolve any remaining mustard and to incorporate any juices on the sheet pan into the sauce.

Tandoori Chicken Cutlets

This recipe needs to marinate overnight.

MAKES 6 SERVINGS

Preparation time: 15 minutes, plus overnight marinating

Cooking time: 25 minutes

3 cloves garlic

1-inch piece fresh ginger

2 fresh green chili peppers

1½ cups fat-free plain yogurt

2 tablespoons tandoori masala spice mix

Juice from 1 lemon

Salt and pepper

6 skinless boneless chicken breasts

1. Crush the garlic, ginger, and chili peppers completely.
2. Mix the garlic mixture with the yogurt, spice mix, lemon juice, salt, and pepper until thoroughly combined and smooth.
3. Score the chicken breasts and coat them with the yogurt mixture, cover, then place in refrigerator to marinate overnight.
4. The next day, remove the chicken from the marinade and discard the remaining marinade. Place the breasts in an oven-proof dish in a single layer.
5. Bake the breasts in a preheated 400°F oven for 20 minutes, or until a thermometer inserted into the thickest part of the chicken registers 170°. Turn the oven up to Broil and brown chicken for an additional 5 minutes before serving.

Lemon Chicken

MAKES 4 SERVINGS

Preparation time: 20 minutes

Cooking time: 35 minutes

1 pound 5 ounces boneless, skinless chicken breasts

1 medium onion, sliced

2 cloves garlic, chopped

½ tablespoon finely chopped fresh ginger

Juice and zest from 2 lemons

2 tablespoons soy sauce

½ cup + 2 tablespoons water

2 bay leaves, 3 sprigs fresh thyme, and 4 sprigs fresh parsley
   (including stalks) tied up with kitchen string

1 pinch cinnamon

1 pinch ground ginger

Salt and pepper

1. Cut the meat into 1-inch cubes.
2. Heat a large nonstick pan with a lid over medium heat. Add the onion, garlic, and fresh ginger and cook, covered, for 3 to 4 minutes.
3. Turn heat to high, uncover the pan, add the chicken, and stir continuously for 2 minutes with a spatula until brown.
4. Add the lemon juice, soy sauce, and water.
5. Add the fresh herbs, cinnamon, ground ginger, and lemon zest.
6. Reduce the heat, season to taste with salt and pepper, and simmer, covered, for 30 minutes. Serve hot.

Turkey and Chicken Rolls

MAKES 2 SERVINGS

Preparation time: 5 minutes

2 slices low-sodium turkey deli meat
2 slices low-sodium chicken deli meat
4 teaspoons fat-free cream cheese
Garlic and herbs to taste

1. Separate the individual slices of deli meat and place on a plate.
2. In a bowl, mix the cream cheese with the garlic and herbs.
3. Spread this mixture on each slice of deli meat and roll up into individual rolls.
4. Cut each roll into 6 pieces and serve.

———————— *Fish Recipes* ————————

Steamed Sole

MAKES 4 SERVINGS

Preparation time: 10 minutes

Cooking time: 10 minutes

2 pounds sole fillets
1 fresh lemon, cut in quarters
2 tablespoons chopped fresh parsley
Salt and pepper

1. Cut the fish into 8 pieces and pat dry with a paper towel. Place the fish on a plate.
2. Fill a steamer with ¾ inch of water and bring to a boil. Place the plate with fish in the steamer and cook for 10 minutes.
3. Top the fish with lemon, chopped parsley, salt, and pepper and serve the fish with its juices. Serve immediately.

Cod Fillets in Mussel Broth

MAKES 4 SERVINGS
Preparation time: 15 minutes
Cooking time: 25 minutes

Four 5-ounce cod fillets
1 large onion, sliced
1 pound fresh mussels, rinsed and well scrubbed
½ cup dry white wine
Juice from 1 fresh lemon
Salt
Lemon wedges, for garnish

1. Preheat oven to 450°F.
2. Wash the cod and place in a large baking dish, topped with the sliced onion.
3. Place the cod in the oven, uncovered, to bake for 20 minutes.
4. Discard any mussels with shells that are open or broken and that do not close when tapped.
5. Place the cleaned mussels in a pot with a lid and add the wine. Cover the pot and cook over high heat until the liquid comes to a boil. Reduce heat to a simmer, and cook for about 4 to 5 minutes, just until the mussels open. During cooking, shake the pot so the mussels can cook evenly. Discard any unopened mussels. Drain and save the cooking liquid from the mussels.
6. Add the lemon juice to the cooking liquid from the mussels and strain it well.
7. Remove the cod dish from the oven and pour the mussel liquid over the fish. Season with pepper and return the fish to the oven to continue baking, uncovered.
8. Shell the mussels and add them to the cod for the last 5 minutes of cooking time along with 2 tablespoons of water and a dash of salt.

9. Discard the juices from the pan before serving. Serve with fresh lemon wedges.

The next three recipes—Grilled Fish, Baked Fish, and Poached Fish—can be made with many different kinds of fish, such as salmon, cod, catfish, halibut, flounder, sea bass, tuna, or swordfish.

Serve any leftovers with Green Mayonnaise (page 179).

Grilled Fish

MAKES 4 SERVINGS
Preparation time: 15 minutes
Cooking time: 10 minutes

Four 6-ounce boneless fish fillets
¼ teaspoon fresh dill *or* a pinch dried dill
¼ teaspoon fresh tarragon *or* a pinch dried tarragon
½ small onion, chopped
Salt and pepper
1 fresh lemon, cut into 4 wedges

1. Heat the grill, or preheat oven to 400°F.
2. Wash and pat the fillets dry with a paper towel.
3. Sprinkle the herbs and chopped onions on the fish and season with pepper.
4. Place the fish either on the grill (with the rack lightly oiled with vegetable oil), or in the oven until cooked to your liking, about 10 minutes.
5. Season with salt after cooking. Serve with fresh lemon wedges.

Baked Fish

MAKES 4 SERVINGS

Preparation time: 5 minutes

Cooking time: 15 minutes

Four 6-ounce fish fillets

½ cup dry white wine

Salt and pepper

4 fresh sprigs dill *or* 1 teaspoon dried dill

1 fresh lemon, cut into 4 wedges

1. Preheat oven to 375°F.
2. Wash and pat the fish dry with paper towels.
3. Place the fish skin side down in a clear baking dish.
4. Add the wine and pepper. Place dill on each fillet.
5. Bake until the fish is just opaque in the center, about 15 minutes.
6. Lightly salt the fish, and discard the juice from the pan. Serve with fresh lemon wedges.

Poached Fish

MAKES 6 SERVINGS

Preparation time: 10 minutes

Cooking time: 5 minutes

⅓ cup water

⅓ cup dry white wine

1 shallot, sliced

4 fresh parsley sprigs *or* 1 teaspoon dried parsley

2 teaspoons fresh thyme *or* 1 teaspoon dried thyme

Six 6-ounce fish fillets

1 fresh lemon, cut into 4 wedges

1. Combine the water, wine, sliced shallot, parsley, and thyme in a large skillet with a lid.
2. Place the salmon fillets in the skillet, skin side down.
3. Cover tightly and simmer on a medium-high heat for about 5 minutes.
4. Remove from the heat and allow to stand, covered, for 5 minutes.
5. Discard the pan juices and serve with lemon wedges.

Baked Salmon Parcel

MAKES 4 SERVINGS

Preparation time: 15 minutes

Cooking time: 20 minutes

Four 6-ounce salmon steaks cut from the middle of the fish
1 teaspoon chopped fresh dill *or* ½ teaspoon dried dill
Juice from 1 lemon
Salt and pepper
1 leek and 1 onion, sliced, for flavor only; discard after cooking

1. Preheat oven to 400°F.
2. Cover a baking sheet with a piece of aluminum foil large enough to enclose the fish.
3. Place the salmon steaks in a single layer on the foil-covered baking sheet and sprinkle with dill, lemon juice, salt, and pepper.
4. Add the onion and leek slices for flavoring; discard after cooking during the Attack diet stage.
5. Bring the edges of the foil up around the salmon to form a packet and tightly seal the seams to capture the liquid produced during cooking.
6. Bake for 20 minutes, or less, according to your taste. Serve immediately.

Mussels *Marinières*

The French word marinière *translates as "seaman-style." In this simple style of preparation, the mussels are cooked with a little white wine, onions, and herbs.*

MAKES 2 SERVINGS; CAN BE DOUBLED TO MAKE 4 SERVINGS

Preparation time: 15 minutes

Cooking time: 5 minutes

2 pounds medium-size mussels, rinsed and well washed

½ medium onion, sliced

1 cup chopped parsley

2 cloves garlic, chopped

¼ teaspoon fresh thyme *or* pinch dried thyme

1 bay leaf

1 cup dry white wine

¼ teaspoon ground pepper

¼ teaspoon salt

1. Place the cleaned mussels in a pot with a lid. Discard any shells that are open or broken and that do not close when tapped, and add the onion, parsley, garlic, thyme, bay leaf, wine, and pepper.
2. Cover the pot and cook over a high heat until the liquid comes to a boil.
3. Reduce the heat to a simmer and cook for about 4 to 5 minutes, until the mussels open. During cooking, shake the pot so the mussels can cook evenly. Discard any unopened mussels.
4. Place the mussels on a platter with the juice. Add salt to the juice and serve.

Crab-Stuffed Eggs

MAKES 4 SERVINGS

Preparation time: 15 minutes

Cooking time: 12 minutes (for the hard-boiled eggs)

1½ pounds fresh crabmeat, cartilage removed

1 recipe Classic Mayonnaise (page 178)

4 hard-boiled eggs

1. In a large bowl, mix the mayonnaise with the crabmeat.
2. Cut the eggs in half lengthwise and scoop out the yolks. Save the yolks for another purpose, such as Oil-Free Mayonnaise (page 179).
3. Fill the egg whites with the crabmeat mixture. Serve immediately or cover and refrigerate until ready to serve.

Note: Crab can be replaced with prawns, shrimp, or tuna.

Scallops Gratin

MAKES 4 SERVINGS

Preparation time: 25 minutes

Cooking time: 30 minutes

2 hard-boiled eggs

4 large scallops

4 cups water

3 tablespoons wine vinegar

1 pound mussels, rinsed and well washed

¼ cup dry white wine

1 shallot, chopped

¼ cup fresh parsley, chopped *or* 1 tablespoon dried parsley

¼ pound shrimp, peeled, deveined, and rinsed

1. Preheat oven to 400°F.
2. Mash the hard-boiled eggs.
3. Place scallops, water, and vinegar in a saucepan and cook for 7 minutes over medium heat.
4. Discard any mussels that are open or broken and that do not close when tapped. Place the cleaned mussels in a lidded pot and add the wine.
5. Cover the pot and cook over high heat until the liquid comes to a boil. Reduce the heat to a simmer and cook for about 4 to 5 minutes, until the mussels open. During cooking, shake the pot so the mussels can cook evenly. Discard any unopened mussels. Strain the liquid from the mussels and save. Remove the mussels from their shells.
6. Mix together the hard-boiled eggs, chopped shallots, parsley, shelled mussels, and shrimp.
7. Cut the scallops into large cubes and add them to the mixture.
8. Add half of the reserved mussel juice to the mixture.
9. Put the mixture in four 6-ounce ramekins.
10. Place the ramekins on a sheet tray and bake for 15 minutes.

Shrimp with Mayonnaise

MAKES 2 SERVINGS; CAN BE DOUBLED TO MAKE 4 SERVINGS
Preparation time: 15 minutes, plus 20 minutes for the shrimp to cool
Cooking time: 5 minutes

4 cups water
2 pounds shrimp, peeled, deveined, and rinsed
3 tablespoons vinegar
1 recipe Classic Mayonnaise (page 178)

1. Fill a large pot with water and bring to a boil. Place the shrimp in boiling water with the vinegar and cook until pink, about 5 minutes.
2. Let shrimp cool in the cooking water for 20 minutes.
3. Drain and serve with the mayonnaise.

Shrimp Sautéed in Herbs

MAKES 2 SERVINGS; CAN BE DOUBLED TO MAKE 4 SERVINGS

Preparation time: 10 minutes

Cooking time: 5 minutes

2 pounds shrimp, peeled, deveined, and rinsed

4 garlic cloves, crushed

½ cup chopped fresh parsley

¼ cup dry white wine

1 fresh lemon, cut in half

1. Heat a nonstick frying pan on medium heat and add the shrimp, garlic, parsley, and white wine.
2. Sauté over medium high heat until the shrimp are pink, about 5 minutes. Serve with fresh lemon.

Note: During the Cruise phase, add vegetables such as mushrooms, asparagus tips, or tomatoes.

Bouillabaisse

MAKES 4 TO 6 SERVINGS
Preparation time: 15 minutes
Cooking time: 45 minutes

1 pound leeks, cleaned and chopped

1 large yellow onion, finely chopped

3 ripe tomatoes, finely chopped

4 garlic cloves, crushed

½ bunch fresh parsley, chopped

2 fennel stalks

1 low-sodium fish bouillon cube

1 cup water

3 bay leaves

2 sprigs fresh thyme *or* 1 teaspoon dried thyme

1 teaspoon fresh basil *or* ½ teaspoon dried basil

1 pound 10 ounces white fish fillet such as cod, flounder, halibut, or scallops

Salt and pepper to taste

1 cup more water for Step 1

12 cups boiling water for Step 2

5 to 6 generous pinches saffron

2 pounds 3 ounces shellfish with shells, such as crawfish, lobster, crab, mussels, or shrimp

1. In a large pot over medium low heat, cook leeks, onions, tomatoes, garlic, parsley, fennel, fish bouillon cube, 1 cup water, bay leaves, thyme, basil, salt, and pepper for 15 minutes.
2. Add 12 cups of boiling water and simmer for an additional 15 minutes.
3. Take the pot off the heat and remove the fennel stalks.
4. Strain the mixture through a colander lined with cheesecloth. Save the fish broth and place in a pot.

5. Add the saffron to the fish broth. Season to taste with salt and pepper.
6. Bring the fish broth to a boil. Reduce the heat to a simmer and poach the fish in the broth, starting first with the firm-fleshed pieces, for about 6 minutes. Remove the fish and set aside.
7. Poach the shellfish in the fish broth until cooked, about 5 minutes. Place everything in a large serving bowl and serve hot.

Note: When serving, do not forget to provide plenty of napkins and extra bowls for the shells.

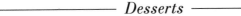

— *Desserts* —

Coffee, Vanilla, or Chocolate Crème

MAKES 4 SERVINGS

Preparation time: 10 minutes plus a minimum of 3 hours chilling time
Cooking time: 10 minutes

3 egg yolks
⅛ teaspoon cornstarch
1 cup nonfat milk
Flavoring, one of the following: 1 teaspoon instant coffee, *or*
    1 teaspoon natural unsweetened cocoa powder dissolved
    in water, *or* the seeds from 1 vanilla pod mixed with a few
    drops vanilla extract
Zero-calorie sweetener to taste

1. Mix the egg yolks with the cornstarch and beat until smooth.
2. Pour the milk into a saucepan and add the flavoring.
3. Warm the milk over low heat just to the boiling point. Remove from the heat.
4. Add the warmed milk mixture to the egg yolks and cornstarch mixture and beat until incorporated.

5. Pour the mixture into the saucepan and place over low heat, stirring constantly with a wooden spoon until the mixture thickens and coats the back of the spoon, about 4 to 5 minutes. Remove from the heat as soon as this occurs.

6. If desired, add sweetener to taste.

7. Pour the crème into a large dish or 4 individual 4-ounce ramekins.

8. Cover the crème and place in the refrigerator for at least 3 hours. Serve very cold.

Note: This recipe can be made into ice cream: let the mixture chill and follow the manufacturer's instructions for your specific ice cream maker.

Custard

MAKES 6 SERVINGS

Preparation time: 20 minutes plus a minimum of 2 hours 30 minutes chilling time

Cooking time: 35 minutes

5 eggs
1 fresh vanilla pod, split lengthwise
1½ cups nonfat milk
1 tablespoon vanilla extract
1 teaspoon freshly ground nutmeg, plus a pinch for garnish

1. Preheat oven to 300°F.

2. In a large heatproof bowl, beat the eggs until smooth.

3. Pour the milk into a medium saucepan. Scrape out the inside of the vanilla pod and add the seeds and the bean to the milk.

4. Over low heat, heat the milk until small bubbles appear around the edge of the pan. Do not let the milk boil.

5. Remove the vanilla pod and slowly pour the hot milk over the eggs, stirring constantly.

6. Add the vanilla extract and 1 teaspoon ground nutmeg.
7. Pour the mixture into 6 individual ramekins.
8. Sprinkle each with additional grated nutmeg.
9. Place the ramekins in a large baking pan and fill the pan with boiling water three-quarters of the way up the sides of the ramekins.
10. Bake for 30 to 35 minutes.
11. Allow the custards to cool in the pan for 30 minutes and place in the refrigerator covered for 2 hours before serving.

Dukan Floating Island

MAKES 4 SERVINGS

Preparation time: 15 minutes plus a minimum of 3 hours chilling time

Cooking time: 15 minutes

4 raw eggs *or* 4 pasteurized eggs, separated
2 cups nonfat milk
1 vanilla pod, split lengthwise
Zero-calorie sweetener to taste

1. In a mixing bowl, beat the egg whites until they form soft but firm peaks.
2. In a saucepan, bring the milk and the vanilla pod to a gentle boil.
3. With a ladle, carefully spoon out 4 to 6 snowball-size portions of the egg whites and drop them into the hot milk. They will swell up.
4. Turn them over in the warm milk, remove them, with a slotted spoon, and let them drain on a plate.
5. Beat the egg yolks and gradually whisk in the warm milk and vanilla mixture.
6. Put the egg yolk and milk mixture back in the saucepan over low heat, stirring constantly.

7. When the mixture starts to thicken and the custard coats the back of a wooden spoon, quickly remove it from the heat or it will curdle.

8. Sweeten to taste.

9. Put the mixture in a glass bowl and let it cool for 10 minutes. Place the egg white snowballs delicately on the surface.

10. Cover and refrigerate for 3 hours and serve chilled.

Note: When beating the egg whites, you can use a dash of cream of tartar to make it easier to form soft peaks.

Recipes for the Cruise Phase: Proteins + Vegetables

—————— *Vegetable Recipes* ——————

· Cauliflower Gratin

MAKES 4 SERVINGS

Preparation time: 20 minutes

Cooking time: 30 minutes

1 head cauliflower, roughly chopped

½ pound 93% lean ground beef

Salt and pepper to taste

2 onions, sliced

2 cloves garlic, minced

1 teaspoon fresh parsley

1 cup fat-free shredded cheddar cheese

1. Preheat oven to 350°F.
2. Place cauliflower in a large pot and bring to a boil. Cover, reduce heat to a simmer, and cook for 5 minutes. Drain cauliflower and purée in a food processor until the consistency of mashed potatoes.
3. Heat a large heavy-bottomed skillet over medium heat and cook the ground beef until browned, about 5 minutes. Drain off any excess fat. Season with salt and pepper.
4. Place the browned ground beef into an ovenproof baking dish and top with the onion, garlic, and parsley. Top with the cauliflower purée.
5. Sprinkle the cauliflower purée with fat-free shredded cheddar cheese and bake for 20 minutes.

Mushroom Fricassee

MAKES 4 SERVINGS AS A SIDE DISH

Preparation time: 15 minutes

Cooking time: 20 minutes

1 cup chopped onions
½ cup low-sodium chicken broth
4 cups sliced fresh mushrooms, any variety, cleaned and stems removed
1 clove garlic, diced
¼ cup chopped fresh parsley
Salt and pepper

1. In a nonstick frying pan over medium heat, cook the chopped onions in the broth until they are caramel colored.
2. Add the mushrooms to the pan and cook slowly over low heat, uncovered, for 10 minutes.
3. Add garlic, parsley, salt, and pepper.

Serve hot with meat or poultry.

Stuffed Mushrooms

MAKES 20 HORS D'OEUVRES OR CAN BE SERVED
AS AN APPETIZER

Preparation time: 25 minutes

Cooking time: 40 minutes

20 large portobello mushrooms
2 cloves garlic, chopped
½ cup chopped fresh parsley
2 teaspoons nonfat milk
Salt and pepper

1. Preheat oven to 400°F.
2. Remove the stems from the mushrooms and reserve. Most portobellos that you buy are very clean, but if the mushrooms are at all dirty, brush them with a small kitchen brush or paper towel to remove the dirt.
3. Chop the stems of the mushrooms, place in a large bowl, and add the garlic, parsley, nonfat milk, salt, and pepper.
4. Cook this stem mixture in a nonstick frying pan on medium heat for about 10 minutes.
5. Meanwhile, bake the mushroom caps stem side down for 10 minutes.
6. Fill the hollow mushroom caps with the cooked stuffing and return them to the oven to bake for 20 minutes.

Note: This recipe can be easily halved or quartered.

Spinach with White Sauce

This recipe is good served with hard-boiled eggs cut into halves,
or with meat or poultry.

MAKES 6 SERVINGS AS A SIDE DISH
Preparation time: 20 minutes
Cooking time: 30 minutes

1 pound fresh spinach leaves, washed
4 cups lightly salted water
1 recipe White Sauce (page 182)

1. Preheat oven to 350°F.
2. Bring the water to boil in a large pot and cook the spinach for 5 minutes.
3. Drain the spinach completely and crush the leaves with a slotted spoon.
4. Put the spinach in an ovenproof dish, pour the White Sauce over the spinach, and bake for 20 minutes.

Cucumbers—Served Hot or Cold

To prepare hot
MAKES 4 SERVINGS AS SIDE DISH;
MAKES 2 SERVINGS AS AN APPETIZER
Preparation time: 15 minutes
Cooking time: 10 minutes

2 cucumbers, peeled and sliced
¼ cup vinegar
Salt to taste
1 recipe White Sauce (page 182)

1. Put the peeled and sliced cucumbers in a saucepan and cover with water.

2. Add the vinegar and cook for 10 minutes over high heat.

3. Add salt to taste.

4. Drain the cucumbers and serve with the White Sauce.

To prepare cold

MAKES 4 SERVINGS AS SIDE DISH;

MAKES 2 SERVINGS AS AN APPETIZER

Preparation time: 15 minutes, plus 1 hour for the cucumbers to drain

2 cucumbers, peeled

3 tablespoons fat-free sour cream

2 teaspoons Dijon mustard

2 teaspoons minced garlic

1. Cut the cucumbers in half lengthwise. Scrape out the seeds with a spoon.

2. Slice the cucumbers and place in a colander to drain for an hour.

3. In a medium-size bowl, thoroughly mix the fat-free sour cream, the Dijon mustard, and the minced garlic. Serve the sour cream sauce with the cucumbers.

Green Cabbage Gratin

MAKES 4 SERVINGS

Preparation time: 25 minutes

Cooking time: 30 minutes

1½ pounds green cabbage, washed and coarsely chopped

1 teaspoon salt

1 recipe White Sauce (page 182)

1 egg

1. Preheat oven to 375°F.

2. Bring a large pot of water to a boil and add the cabbage.

3. Cook for 5 minutes on high heat.
4. Add salt and drain the cabbage.
5. Place the cabbage in a baking dish and stir in the White Sauce.
6. Beat the egg and pour it over the cabbage.
7. Bake uncovered for 25 minutes until the top is golden brown.

Note: You can substitute endive for cabbage in this recipe.

Butternut Squash Soup

MAKES 10 TO 12 SERVINGS
Preparation time: 30 minutes
Cooking time: 30 minutes

1 butternut squash, seeds removed, peeled, and cut into large pieces
1 large onion, chopped
1 apple, peeled, seeds and core removed
3 quarts low-sodium chicken broth
Salt and pepper
1 tablespoon curry powder
½ cup fat-free sour cream *or* fat-free plain yogurt

1. Put the squash, onion, apple, and chicken broth in a large pot and cook for 20 to 30 minutes, until the squash is very soft.
2. Purée the soup in batches in a blender and return to the pot.
3. Add the salt, pepper, and curry powder and mix in the sour cream or yogurt until thoroughly combined.

Note: This soup can be served hot or cold. If reheating, do not allow the soup to boil.

Miracle Soup

This soup is extremely filling and is highly recommended for people who arrive home starving after a long day at work because they only ate a tiny lunch or skipped lunch altogether. For those of you who can't resist snacking on something right away, try one bowl of this soup, served hot, and you will find that these cravings disappear and that you are able to comfortably wait for your dinner without overeating.

MAKES 8 TO 10 SERVINGS
Preparation time: 25 minutes
Cooking time: 20 minutes

4 cloves garlic, chopped
6 large onions, chopped
1 large head of cabbage, cored and sliced
6 carrots, peeled and sliced
2 green peppers, seeds removed and chopped
1 bunch of celery, sliced
One 35-ounce can peeled tomatoes
3 low-sodium beef bouillon cubes
3 low-sodium chicken bouillon cubes

1. Put the prepared garlic, onions, cabbage, carrots, green peppers, celery, and tomatoes in a soup pot and cover with water.
2. Add the beef and chicken bouillon cubes.
3. Bring the soup to a boil and continue cooking at a boil for 10 minutes. Reduce the heat to a simmer and continue cooking until the vegetables are tender, about 10 additional minutes.

Note: The soup will keep, covered, in the refrigerator for 3 days.

Zucchini Velouté

Velouté *means "velvety," a perfect description for this smooth and velvety puréed soup.*

MAKES 6 TO 8 SERVINGS
Preparation time: 20 minutes
Cooking time: 20 to 30 minutes

4 large zucchini, washed and sliced
1 large onion, sliced
1 carrot, peeled and sliced
1 turnip, peeled and sliced
2 quarts low-sodium beef broth

1. Place the zucchini, onion, carrot, and turnip in a large pot and cover with the beef broth.
2. Bring the broth to a simmer and cook for 20 to 30 minutes.
3. Pour the soup into a blender and purée until smooth, about 1 minute. Serve hot.

———— *Protein + Vegetable Recipes* ————

Herbed Chicken Salad

MAKES 2 SERVINGS

Preparation time: 25 minutes

Cooking time: 10 minutes

1 boneless skinless chicken breast

1 cup low-sodium chicken broth

¾ cup fat-free plain yogurt

1 clove garlic, chopped

1 teaspoon Dijon mustard

1 tablespoon chopped fresh parsley

1 tablespoon chopped fresh chives

Salt and black pepper

1⅓ cups button mushrooms, cleaned and cut into small cubes

1 bunch radishes, trimmed and cut into small cubes

2 small sour, half-sour, or French cornichon pickles, sliced

1. Place chicken breast and chicken broth in a small skillet with a lid. Bring to a boil, reduce heat to a simmer, cover, and cook for 10 minutes. Remove chicken from poaching liquid, let cool, and cut into strips.

2. In a large bowl, mix together the yogurt, garlic, mustard, parsley, chives, salt, and pepper.

3. Add the cubed mushrooms and radishes, the chicken, and the pickles and mix until combined. Refrigerate until served.

Three-Pepper Tuna

MAKES 4 SERVINGS

Preparation time: 35 minutes, plus 2 to 3 hours for marinating

Cooking time: 25 minutes

1 red pepper

1 green pepper

1 yellow pepper

1 teaspoon vegetable oil

1 pound 9 ounces tuna steaks

Salt and white pepper

Juice of 1 lemon

2 cloves garlic, crushed

1. Place the peppers under a preheated broiler for 5 minutes, remove from the broiler, and immediately place in a plastic bag for 10 minutes to facilitate peeling.

2. When the peppers are cool, peel, remove the seeds, and cut into strips.

3. Heat a heavy-bottomed skillet over medium heat. Add the teaspoon of oil to the skillet and then wipe the skillet with a paper towel. Add the peppers and cook until the peppers are tender, about 5 to 10 minutes. Add a little water to the bottom of the pan if the peppers begin to stick.

4. Place the tuna steaks in a steamer over 1 inch of boiling water and cover. Cook for 10 to 15 minutes. Place the tuna in a nonreactive bowl or platter and season with salt and white pepper. Allow it to cool for 30 minutes.

5. Mix together the lemon juice, garlic, and pepper strips and set aside.

6. When the tuna is cool, mix the tuna and the pepper mixture together and marinate in the refrigerator for 2 to 3 hours. Turn the tuna regularly while it is marinating. Serve cold.

Turgloff Beef Kebabs

MAKES 4 SERVINGS

Preparation time: 25 minutes

Cooking time: 25 minutes

1 pound 2 ounces fresh tomatoes, peel and seeds removed,
   chopped
1 clove garlic
Salt and black pepper
1 pound 5 ounces lean beef, cut into 1-inch cubes
1 sweet pepper, cut into 1-inch cubes
1 onion, cut into 1-inch cubes
Juice of 1 lemon
Celery salt
1 teaspoon chopped fresh parsley, for garnish

1. Make the tomato sauce: Place the tomatoes and garlic in a frying pan and bring to a simmer. Cook for 15 minutes.
2. Season the tomato sauce with salt and pepper to taste. Set aside.
3. Place the beef, peppers, and onions on kebab skewers and grill or broil for about 10 minutes, turning once.
4. Remove the beef and vegetables from the skewers, sprinkle with lemon juice, and add some celery salt.
5. Top the kebabs with the tomato sauce.
6. Adjust the seasoning and garnish with chopped parsley.

Chicken Marengo

MAKES 4 SERVINGS

Preparation time: 15 minutes

Cooking time: 40 minutes

1 medium onion, sliced

½ cup of low-sodium chicken broth

2 tomatoes, chopped

¼ teaspoon fresh thyme *or* a pinch dried thyme

Salt and pepper

4 boneless skinless chicken breasts, cut into chunks

½ cup dry white wine

½ cup sliced mushrooms

1. In a nonstick frying pan with a lid, place the sliced onions to cover the bottom and add the chicken broth. Simmer until the onions are golden, about 10 minutes.
2. Add the chopped tomatoes, thyme, pepper, and salt.
3. Place the chicken on the onions and add the wine. Cover and allow to cook over low heat for 20 minutes.
4. Add the sliced mushrooms and cook for an additional 10 minutes.
5. Remove the chicken and set aside. Reduce the excess liquid by rapidly boiling the pan juices uncovered for a few seconds.
6. Pour the pan juices over the chicken and serve.

Mushroom Frittata

MAKES 4 SERVINGS

Preparation time: 15 minutes

Cooking time: 40 minutes

2 cups fresh mushrooms, sliced

2 onions, chopped

5 large eggs

Salt and pepper

1. Preheat oven to 350°F.
2. In nonstick frying pan, sauté the sliced mushrooms and chopped onions for 10 minutes on medium heat.
3. Beat the eggs and add the mushrooms and onions, plus salt and pepper to taste. Pour the mixture into a deep baking dish.
4. Bake covered with foil for 30 minutes.

Dukan Chicken and Herb Omelet Sandwich

This recipe is a fun way to use leftover cooked chicken.

MAKES 1 SERVING

Preparation time: 20 minutes

Cooking time: 10 minutes

2 tablespoons oat bran

1 tablespoon wheat bran

1 teaspoon baking powder

2 tablespoons fat-free plain Greek yogurt

2 eggs + 1 egg white

1 tablespoon fresh chopped parsley

Fresh herbs of your choice, such as basil, mixed herbs, or shallots

2 tablespoons fat-free cream cheese

1 *cooked* boneless, skinless chicken breast, chopped*

*If you do not have any leftover cooked chicken, follow the instructions for poaching uncooked chicken as given in the Herbed Chicken Salad recipe (page 220).

1. In a small bowl, thoroughly mix the oat bran, wheat bran, baking powder, yogurt, 1 whole egg, and the chopped parsley.

2. Place in a 10 × 12-inch microwave-safe dish and microwave on High for 4 minutes.

3. Remove this "bread" from the dish and allow to cool a little before cutting into 2 slices. Toast very lightly in a toaster oven or under the broiler for about 3 minutes, and do not let the bread dry out.

4. In a medium-size bowl, beat the remaining egg, the egg white, and herbs.

5. Heat a small nonstick frying pan over medium heat. Pour the egg mixture into the hot pan and cook without stirring, shaking the pan occasionally until you have an egg "pancake."

6. Fold over the four edges of the "pancake" to make a rectangle.

7. Spread each slice of bread with the cream cheese.

8. Assemble the sandwich by putting the chopped chicken on one slice of bread. Top with the omelet and cover with the second slice of bread.

Dukan Hamburger

MAKES 1 SERVING

Preparation time: 20 minutes

Cooking time: 10 minutes

2 tablespoons oat bran

1 tablespoon wheat bran

1 teaspoon baking powder

2 tablespoons + 1 teaspoon fat-free plain Greek yogurt (divided)

1 egg white

½ pound 93% lean ground beef

1 teaspoon Cajun spices, or to taste

1 tablespoon yellow mustard

2 leaves iceberg lettuce

2 slices tomato

1. In a small bowl, thoroughly mix the oat bran, wheat bran, baking powder, 2 tablespoons of yogurt, and the egg white.

2. Place in a 10 × 12-inch microwave-safe dish and microwave at high setting for 4 minutes.

3. Remove this "bread" from the dish and allow to cool a little before cutting into 2 slices. Toast very lightly in a toaster oven or under the broiler for about 3 minutes, and do not let the bread dry out.

4. Preheat the oven to Broil. Mix together the beef, the Cajun spices, and the 1 teaspoon of Greek yogurt and form into a patty.

5. Broil the patty until cooked to your liking.

6. Spread each slice of "bread" with the mustard.

7. Assemble the sandwich by placing the meat, the lettuce, and the tomatoes slices on one slice of bread and covering them with the second slice of bread.

Lettuce-Wrap Burritos

MAKES 4 SERVINGS

Preparation time: 20 minutes

Cooking time: 45 minutes

2 cloves garlic, crushed

1 medium onion, diced

1 tablespoon water

1½ pounds 93% lean ground beef

1 sweet red pepper, seeded and diced

1 small red chili pepper, chopped*

1 tablespoon low-sodium tomato juice

¾ cup tomato paste

½ cup low-sodium beef broth

8 big leaves iceberg lettuce

4 tablespoons no-sugar-added tomato sauce, store-bought or homemade†

1. Heat a nonstick pan over medium heat. Add the crushed garlic cloves, the diced onion, and 1 tablespoon of water. Cook until the onions and garlic become tender, about 5 minutes.

2. Add the ground beef and stir continuously until cooked to medium, about 5 minutes.

3. Add the sweet pepper, chopped chili pepper, ½ tablespoon tomato juice, tomato paste, and the beef broth to the pan.

4. Reduce the heat to low and simmer for 10 minutes, stirring often.

5. Lay the lettuce leaves on a platter and fill each one with an equal portion of the beef mixture. Add the remaining ½ tablespoon tomato juice and the tomato sauce to the filled lettuce leaves.

*For less heat, discard the seeds and the ribs of the chili pepper. The best chili peppers for this dish are jalapeños.

†Commercial tomato sauce should have no more than 1 gram of sugar per serving.

Dukan Crab Cakes

MAKES 2 SERVINGS, 2 CRAB CAKES PER SERVING

Preparation time: 10 minutes, plus 1 hour for refrigeration
before cooking

Cooking time: 25 minutes

2 egg yolks, divided
1 pound fresh crabmeat, cartilage removed
Juice from ½ fresh lemon
¼ teaspoon ground cumin
¼ teaspoon chopped fresh cilantro
¼ teaspoon turmeric
1 teaspoon powdered ginger
3 tablespoons cornstarch

1. Preheat oven to 350°F.
2. Beat 1 egg yolk.
3. Mix together the crabmeat, lemon juice, cumin, chopped cilantro, turmeric, ginger, cornstarch, and the beaten egg yolk. Let the mixture rest, covered, in the refrigerator for 1 hour.
4. Spray 4 muffin tin cups with nonstick spray. Form the crab mixture into 4 balls and place them in the sprayed muffin cups. Put a little water in the remaining empty cups to keep them from scorching.
5. Beat the second egg yolk and brush it on the crab cakes.
6. Place the muffin tin in the oven and bake the crab cakes for 25 minutes.

Note: In the Cruise phase, serve the crab cakes with tomato slices and lettuce leaves.

Dukan Pizza

MAKES 1 SERVING
Preparation time: 10 minutes
Cooking time: 15 minutes

2 tablespoons oat bran

1 tablespoon wheat bran

3 tablespoons powdered nonfat milk

1 egg

1 egg white

3 tablespoons fat-free cream cheese

1 tablespoon fat-free sour cream

2 to 4 ounces smoked salmon

Salt and pepper

1. Preheat oven to 350°F.
2. In a large bowl combine the oat bran, wheat bran, milk powder, egg, and egg white.
3. Heat a small nonstick pan over medium heat, spread the mixture evenly over the bottom of the pan, and cook on one side for 4 minutes.
4. Turn the pancake onto a cookie sheet covered with parchment paper and bake for 3 minutes.
5. Remove the cookie sheet from the oven and temporarily set aside.
6. In a bowl, mix the fat-free cream cheese and the fat-free sour cream, spread the mixture on top of the pancake, and add pieces of smoked salmon.
7. Return to the oven and bake for an additional 8 minutes.

Note: For variety you can substitute tomatoes and anchovies for the smoked salmon, and fat-free feta cheese and artichokes for the cream cheese. For 2 servings, double the ingredients and use a large nonstick pan or bake on a sheet tray for 10 minutes.

Tofu Kebabs

MAKES 4 SERVINGS

Preparation time: 30 minutes, plus 30 minutes for marinating

Cooking time: 10 minutes

1 pound firm tofu, cut into cubes

1 large red pepper, seeds removed and cut into cubes

2 small zucchini, sliced

½ cup button mushrooms, cut in half

2 tablespoons soy sauce

2 teaspoons grated fresh ginger

1 clove garlic, crushed

1 small fresh chili pepper, such as jalapeño, finely chopped*

1. Thread the cubed tofu and red peppers, the sliced zucchini, and the halved mushrooms in alternating order onto 8 skewers. If you are using wooden skewers, soak them in water for at least 15 minutes to prevent burning.
2. Lay the skewers in a large baking dish in a single layer.
3. In a small bowl, thoroughly combine the soy sauce, grated ginger, the crushed garlic, and the chopped chili pepper.
4. Pour this sauce over the kebabs and set aside, covered, for 30 minutes to marinate at room temperature.
5. Remove the skewers from the marinade, reserving the extra liquid. Cook the skewers on a hot grill or under the broiler, basting often with extra marinade.
6. Cook until the tofu is browned, about 10 minutes.

Serve with a tomato salad.

*For less heat, remove the seeds and ribs from the chili pepper.

— *Desserts for the Consolidation Phase* —

The following dessert recipes were tested using Splenda. If you are using another sweetener, the results may vary.

Dukan Muffins

MAKES 4 MUFFINS
Preparation time: 10 minutes
Cooking time: 20 minutes

1 egg

1 egg white

3 tablespoons oat bran

1 teaspoon baking powder

3 tablespoons powdered nonfat milk

2 teaspoons zero-calorie sweetener suitable for baking, such as Splenda

1 teaspoon flavor extract such as vanilla, lemon, cinnamon, coconut, almond, cocoa, or hazelnut

1. Preheat oven to 350°F.
2. Place all the ingredients in a bowl and mix to combine.
3. Pour the mixture into nonstick or silicon muffin tins.
4. Cook for 20 minutes. Let muffins cool in the tins before removing.

Note: If your muffin tin has space for more than 4 muffins, fill the empty spaces with water to prevent the tins from burning.

Oat Bran Chocolate Chip Cookies

MAKES ABOUT 20 COOKIES

Preparation time: 20 minutes, plus 2 hours for the "chocolate bar" to harden

Cooking time: 20 minutes

2 teaspoons Dutch-processed cocoa

1 egg yolk + 1 egg

1 tablespoon zero-calorie sweetener suitable for baking, such as Splenda, divided

3 tablespoons oat bran

¾ cup fat-free plain Greek yogurt

1 tablespoon cornstarch

1 teaspoon baking powder

1 teaspoon vanilla extract

1. In a bowl, mix the cocoa, egg yolk, and 1 teaspoon of the sweetener.

2. Wrap this mixture in plastic wrap and flatten it into a rectangular bar.

3. Put this "chocolate bar" into the freezer for about 2 hours to harden. Once the mixture is firm, chop it into coarse chunks.

4. Preheat oven to 350°F.

5. Put the oat bran and chocolate chunks into a bowl.

6. Add the yogurt, cornstarch, whole egg, baking powder, vanilla extract, and 2 teaspoons of the sweetener.

7. Line a baking sheet with aluminum foil, and with a tablespoon, place small, heaping mounds of mixture on the foil, about 2 inches apart. You will fit 10 to 12 cookies on each sheet. Bake the cookies in two batches for best results.

8. Bake at 350°F for 20 minutes until edges are nicely browned. Let the cookies cool completely before removing from the baking sheet.

Rhubarb Crumble

MAKES 4 SERVINGS

Preparation time: 30 minutes

Cooking time: 50 minutes

1 pound rhubarb, trimmed, washed, and cut into 1-inch pieces

2 teaspoons zero-calorie sweetener suitable for baking, such as
    Splenda

6 tablespoons oat bran

2 tablespoons wheat bran

2 egg whites

2 tablespoons fat-free plain Greek yogurt

1. Preheat oven to 350°F.
2. In a saucepan, cook the rhubarb with the sweetener over low heat for 15 minutes.
3. In a medium-size bowl, mix together the oat bran, wheat bran, egg whites, and yogurt.
4. Cover a baking sheet with parchment paper. Spread the mixture onto the parchment paper.
5. Bake at 350°F for 20 minutes.
6. Remove the baking sheet from the oven and place it on a flat surface. Cut the crumble into pieces, and then break it up further.
7. Return the crumble mixture to the oven and bake for an additional 5 minutes.
8. Put the stewed rhubarb into four 4-ounce ramekins and sprinkle the crumble mixture evenly over each.
9. Place the ramekins in the 350°F oven and bake for about 10 minutes.

Light Cheesecake

MAKES 4 SERVINGS

Preparation time: 10 minutes, plus a minimum of
4 hours 30 minutes to chill
Cooking time: 12 minutes

10 tablespoons fat-free plain Greek yogurt

4 tablespoons cornstarch

4 egg yolks

4 tablespoons lemon juice

2 tablespoons zero-calorie sweetener suitable for baking, such
as Splenda

10 egg whites

1. In a bowl, blend the yogurt, cornstarch, egg yolks, lemon juice, and sweetener until smooth.
2. Whip the egg whites until stiff peaks form, and carefully fold them into the yogurt mixture.
3. Pour the mixture into a 9-inch microwave-safe pan.
4. Microwave for 12 minutes at Medium setting.
5. Cool at room temperature for 30 minutes, then refrigerate for a minimum of 4 hours. Let stand at room temperature for 15 minutes before serving.

One Week of Menus for the Pure Protein Attack Phase

Breakfast—For Every Day of the Week

Coffee or tea with artificial sweetener of your choice

+ choice of: 8 ounces (225 grams) nonfat yogurt *or* nonfat cottage cheese

+ choice of: 1 slice turkey, chicken, or low-fat ham; *or* 1 egg; *or* 1 egg Custard; *or* 1 Dukan Oat Bran Galette

---

At 10 a.m. or 11 a.m. (if hungry)

4 ounces (115 grams) nonfat yogurt *or* nonfat cottage cheese

---

At 4 p.m. (if necessary)

4 ounces (115 grams) nonfat yogurt, *or* 1 slice of turkey, *or* both

Lunch and Dinner for Seven Days

Monday

Make enough food for dinner, so you can have it for lunch the next day, or within the next two days.

Lunch	*Dinner*
Hard-boiled Egg with Dukan Herb Mayonnaise	Shrimp Sautéed in Herbs
Barbecue Steak	Tandoori Chicken Cutlets
8 ounces (225 grams) nonfat yogurt	Custard *or* 4 ounces (115 grams) nonfat yogurt

Tuesday

Lunch	*Dinner*
Baked Salmon Parcel	Crab-Stuffed Eggs
Vietnamese Beef	Chicken with Mustard
8 ounces (225 grams)	Custard *or* 4 ounces (115 grams)
nonfat yogurt	nonfat yogurt

Wednesday

Lunch	*Dinner*
Poached Salmon with Fresh Herb Sauce	Hard-boiled Egg with Ravigote Sauce
Roast Chicken with Tarragon and Lemon	Cod Fillet with Mussel Broth
Custard *or* 1 Dukan Oat Bran Galette	Dukan Floating Island *or* 8 ounces (225 grams) nonfat yogurt *or* nonfat ricotta

Thursday

Lunch	*Dinner*
1 slice Smoked Salmon	Scallop Gratin
Chicken with Mustard	Pork Medallions
Chocolate Crème *or* 8 ounces (225 grams) nonfat ricotta	Custard *or* 4 ounces (115 grams) nonfat yogurt

Friday

Lunch	*Dinner*
Steamed Shrimp with Dukan Herb Mayonnaise	Shrimp Sautéed in Herbs
Grilled Swordfish	Tandoori Chicken Cutlets
8 ounces (225 grams) nonfat yogurt *or* nonfat ricotta	Dukan Floating Island *or* 8 ounces (225g) nonfat yogurt

Saturday

Lunch	Dinner
Turkey and Chicken Rolls	Mussels Marinières
Poached Salmon Fillets	Lemon Chicken
Custard *or* 1 Dukan Oat	Dukan Floating Island *or* 8 ounces (225 grams)
Bran Galette	nonfat yogurt *or* nonfat ricotta

Sunday

Lunch	Dinner
Steamed Sole	Poached Fish
Roast Beef	Chicken with Mustard
Coffee Crème *or* Custard	Dukan Floating Island

One Week of Menus for Pure Proteins
Followed by Pure Proteins + Vegetables

The breakfasts, midmorning, and afternoon snacks for the entire week are the same as for the pure protein Attack phase.

Monday

Lunch	Dinner
Smoked Salmon	Crab-Stuffed Eggs
Baked Salmon	Sliced cold Roast Beef with Hunter's Sauce
Custard *or* 1 Dukan Oat	Coffee Crème *or* 8 ounces (225 grams)
Bran Galette	nonfat yogurt

Tuesday

Lunch	*Dinner*
Stuffed Mushrooms	Butternut Squash Soup
Three-Pepper Tuna	Turgloff Beef Kebab
8 ounces (225 grams) nonfat yogurt	Custard

Wednesday

Lunch	*Dinner*
Hard-boiled Eggs with Ravigote Sauce	Shrimp Sautéed in Herbs
Baked Salmon	Chicken with Mustard
Custard *or* 1 Dukan Oat Bran Galette	Dukan Floating Island *or* 8 ounces (225 grams) nonfat ricotta

Thursday

Lunch	*Dinner*
Stuffed Tomatoes	Zucchini Velouté
Dukan Chicken and Herb Omelet Sandwich	Baked Salmon Parcel
Coffee Crème	Custard *or* 4 ounces (115 grams) nonfat yogurt

Friday

Lunch	*Dinner*
Hard-boiled Eggs with Dukan Herb Mayonnaise	Beef Skewers
Vietnamese Beef	Grilled Fish
Dukan Floating Island *or* Custard	8 ounces (225 grams) nonfat yogurt

Saturday

Lunch	*Dinner*
Lettuce Salad with Vinaigrette #2	Cucumbers, Served Hot or Cold
Cauliflower Gratin	Chicken Marengo
Custard *or* 1 Dukan Oat Bran Galette	Vanilla Crème

Sunday

Lunch	*Dinner*
Shrimp Sautéed with Herbs	Poached Salmon with Hollandaise Sauce
Roast Chicken with Tarragon and Lemon	Pork Medallions
Dukan Floating Island	Chocolate Crème *or* Custard

AFTERWORD

The Dukan Diet owes its success to the enthusiasm of users who have benefited from it and have then worked tirelessly to spread the word. More than two hundred websites, forums, and blogs have been set up by anonymous users and volunteers, mostly women, who, without knowing me, became teachers and advocates of my method.

The rights to the book have been acquired by Italian, Korean, Thai, Spanish, Brazilian, Polish, British, and now North American publishers. As much as I understood the success in France, the stir created through the press and forums in other countries took me by surprise.

After the book appeared in other countries, I received many letters from journalists and doctors telling me how much they liked the method and the successful results they had achieved by following it. They all told me that, however French the method may have appeared at the outset, it had not seemed foreign to them.

Moreover the concept of eating as much as you want responds to the way we function most instinctively and naturally. When we are hungry or thirsty, we should eat or drink until we are satisfied—that is, until there is a return to a biological equilibrium. This need is all the more demanding when it is coupled with a desire or a compulsion of a psychological and emotional nature. It is counting calories and restraining our appetite when faced with tempting food that runs counter to nature.

My Final Word on Low-Calorie Diets

Today, after thirty-five years of daily practice as a physician and nutritionist treating excess weight and obesity, I am convinced that one of the reasons why the struggle against weight problems has failed throughout the world is because low-calorie diets don't work.

In theory, low-calorie diets are the most logical of diets, but in practice they are one of the worst. Why is this so? Because they are based on a model that works against the psychology of people who put on weight. Counting calories only takes into account the cold logic of numbers, ignoring anything to do with feelings, emotions, pleasure, and the need to find sensory gratification.

Low-calorie diets tell us that we eat too much, or eat too many things that are bad or too rich. This is true, but it does not explain *why* we do it. And low-calorie diets also say that we will put on weight because we consume too many calories, so if we cut down the number of calories we eat, we will lose weight. We therefore spend our day calculating to make sure we do not go over the number of calories allocated, whether it be 1,800 or 600.

But what happens if people on a low-calorie diet manage to get down to the weight they want? Can we then ask someone who has put on weight because they have always eaten without keeping track of what they eat to suddenly turn into a calorie counter for the rest of their lives?

To defend this counterproductive diet, which goes against nature, its supporters brandish the word *balance*—as in eating a *balanced* diet. But if overweight people were capable of eating a balanced diet, they would never have become overweight. In thirty-five years, I have not met a single person who *wants* to become big, fat, or obese. If women or men become obese, it is because they were unable to resist eating. Asking such individuals to eat only 900 calories a day will simply add to their confusion and suffering.

Low-calorie diets are doomed to fail, but the people who still use them do not want to acknowledge their failure. Moreover, by definition, the recommendation to cut down and count calories makes any hope of stabilizing the weight achieved impossible. The only exception is the Weight

Watchers method, but it is not the diet itself that is innovative and effective; it is the support of Weight Watchers meetings, which at the time were a real revolution. Weight Watchers are, to my mind, the only ones who can claim to have slowed down the increase in weight problems in the world, until the availability of daily Internet coaching.

However, low-calorie diets without any real monitoring are almost automatically doomed to failure. And I hope that it will be pressure from the very people who actually follow diets that rely on counting calories that will bring about their end.

DAILY INTERACTIVE AND PERSONALIZED MONITORING ON THE INTERNET

A Major, Decisive Advance in Fighting the World's Weight Problems

Several large international studies have shown that one of the major keys to success in the fight against excess weight is for the person trying to slim to be monitored and supervised by a health professional.

Wherever monitoring has been combined with a high-quality diet program, the results obtained have been significantly better, both for losing weight as well as for stabilizing it over the medium term. The only problem is the mathematical impossibility of recruiting millions of nutritionists throughout the world to participate.

Not All Coaching Sites Are Effective

Since the late 1990s, many websites have been set up that offer weight loss coaching based on a program of healthy eating and exercise.

As chairman of an international association that fights against weight problems, I was invited by its American members to see the best of what was happening in this promising field. I met my counterparts in the United States and, with them, looked in the tiniest detail at the largest American coaching websites. I met some of their promoters and their top public relations professionals.

Together we examined the most popular sites' home pages. Their advertising banners offered "personalized, interactive" coaching delivered by professionals.

In fact, we found nothing of the sort. Not a single coaching website was either personalized, let alone interactive. All we ever found was a standardized method cut up and served in chunks to subscribers. These websites certainly have the means to send their subscribers every day a stream of well-presented information of exceptional quality, recipes, exercises, and tips, but they offered *nothing whatsoever addressed to a single individual user.*

So, for example, a husband and wife joining on the same day will receive the same instructions regardless of their difference in age, gender, and weight.

Moreover, what was the point of these instructions and this information if the people giving them out could not then assess the results? The essential feature of coaching and monitoring is precisely that you can come and tell your doctor: "I've followed your instructions to the letter and I've succeeded—Mission Accomplished!"

What Is the Ideal Coaching Site?

Back home in France, I made up my mind to set up a coaching website as I imagined it should be: *a site combining means, weapons, and appeal and capable of working as well as a nutritionist dealing directly with one of his or her patients, but able to offer this service to dozens, hundreds, thousands, and millions of overweight or obese people.*

To achieve objectives, this site would have to be capable of delivering:

- *A professional service.* One that is devised and coordinated by a doctor
- *A personalized service.* One that enables the person offering motivation and instruction to know exactly whom they are talking to and what that person's needs are
- *An interactive service.* One that establishes a feedback dialogue rather than a monologue
- *A daily service.*

Between 2000 and 2004, I worked with a team of thirty-two doctors and three artificial intelligence and Internet technology wizards to create a book written for a single overweight reader—based on an Internet questionnaire of 154 queries—an exploration and analysis of the reader's own weight situation, with a unique solution for losing weight created especially for that person.

I felt it was possible to integrate this invaluable expertise with coaching, and in so doing to give coaching the very essence of what monitoring is—that is, direct communication. This means that the coach can say to the person being coached:

"You know who I am, and I know who you are and what you need, day after day, so you can reach your goal as quickly as possible and with the least possible frustration."

I embarked on this new project with the firm belief that if I achieved my ends, we would at long last have a new weapon that might stand a chance of taking on our runaway weight problem epidemic.

So I got my team of thirty-two doctors and three IT specialists together again. The expertise previously acquired was an enormous help, but the constraints of coaching turned out to be even more demanding. I wanted a system that would allow me to monitor my subscribers on a daily basis, adapting my program to the jungle of their temptations, their traveling, their illnesses, their business lunches, their stresses and weaknesses, as well as their sudden bursts of motivation.

It was particularly important to me that the counselor could receive the subscriber's report every evening. To my mind, this was the only way of knowing if and how the subscriber had followed my instructions, the only way of being able to react, put right, applaud, and gently reprimand day after day, pound after pound, and keep people on track toward their True Weight.

The Next Generation: Real Online Coaching

To do this, we created and patented a new way of communicating, the daily to and fro e-mail system, which works like an interactive loop. It allows me to send out my instructions to each user every morning and for them to send me back their report every evening, which is indispensable for giving them my instructions for the following morning.

This daily interactive monitoring looks after the subscriber from their very first day of the Attack Phase and then never, ever abandons them.

However, I did not want monitoring to stop with Permanent Stabilization, as only in this phase is it possible to know whether the weight loss achieved is lasting: it has been confirmed medically that people who once in their lifetime have gained more than 18 pounds will have altered their natural set point, and that the only way for them not to put weight back on is to adopt protective measures that are as painless as possible but permanent.

I had for a long time been convinced from my work with overweight patients that the vast majority of them had gained their weight because of their natural tendency to cope with life's difficulties by consoling themselves with food. And it is precisely during such difficult moments that overweight individuals have the most need of a reassuring presence and confident guidelines to help them shore up a positive self-image and self-esteem, so vital if they are to persevere.

Along with the daily to and fro e-mails, I decided to deliver a full 1-hour chat session live every day during which I would personally answer the questions that the men and women being coached ask themselves. Nine times out of ten, they already know the answer themselves, but what actually counts is asking the question, being listened to, and being able to lean upon an outside source of willpower.

Stagnation: The First Cause of Failure in a Diet

In the Dukan Diet, as in any battle, there is a tricky moment when the risk of failure is greater than at any other time, and it occurs in Phase 2, the Cruise phase.

> I lose a pound and a half, then I put a pound or so back on the next day. It all comes back, then it goes again and nothing is working. I am getting desperate, doctor, what should I do?

It is these high-risk moments when their effort is not being rewarded that my patients call their "stagnation."

There are many different reasons for stagnation. To start with, there are people who make mistakes with their diet without realizing it or without specifying it in their evening reports. There are women about to have their period who retain enough water to conceal the weight they have lost. Others take in too much salt or do not drink enough water or drink too much sparkling water with a high sodium content. Then there are people who take anti-inflammatory drugs for arthritis or back pain and those on antidepressants or tranquilizers.

There are also people who, having followed so many diets, have lost and regained so much weight that their metabolism now requires far less energy and their body has become resistant to dieting. Then there are those people who become constipated when dieting and who for a short time gain weight as they are not eliminating sufficiently. Perimenopausal women are at the time in their lives when the risk of weight gain is the highest because of a slowdown in their metabolism. Lastly, the reason for the longest and most resistant stagnation is an underactive thyroid, which must be quickly diagnosed and treated.

And it is especially *here,* during these times when the risk of giving up is high, that a listening ear and a reassuring voice are welcome. Coaching and personalized monitoring find their true vocation here. The reason for stagnation has to be identified, explained, understood, and acknowledged, and everything must be put in place to get the wheels of the weight loss machine turning again.

Return to the Attack phase for a few days, increase or reduce fluid intake according to your individual needs; stop eating oversalty foods for the time being; be more physically active; add a 20-, 30-, 40-, 50-, or 60-minute walk; correct constipation with a gentle laxative or stool softener, or by drinking mineral water rich in magnesium on an empty stomach; add some stomach muscle toning sessions.

During a period of weight loss stagnation you have to learn how to tame the passing time and make it your friend. You have to realize that not *gaining* weight is in itself a feat. Giving in and eating what you shouldn't allows your body to regain the upper hand at the very moment when it was so close to giving up and relinquishing more pounds!

Eat pure proteins and nothing else for three days and afterward come back in two days' time after weighing yourself with some good news.

This is the sort of message someone who is having doubts and is succumbing to temptation expects: a promise, a stage, a milestone, hope, and a voice that is both assertive and reassuring.

Weight, Civilization, and Happiness

Being overweight is a sickness of our civilization, and I set up my interactive website because I firmly believe that the Internet holds the future for our fight against weight problems

I have confidence in the Dukan Diet. I have tested it thoroughly and on many patients. Millions of people have lost weight by reading the book you are holding, and many of them have stabilized their weight.

Unfortunately, too many other people have not succeeded. Some of my readers were not sufficiently motivated to even get started, others stopped partway through, and far too many put weight back on again after losing it.

To score a real and wide-ranging victory in the war against weight problems, having a method that works is not enough. We need a method that works and that people follow . . . right to the very end.

Losing weight is seldom simple or easy. For the vast majority of people, it is an ordeal. Here is not the time or place to tell you about my theory of happiness and what it takes to understand it and make it happen. My theory is born out of close contact with so many of my patients who talk to me openly about their lives, knowing that I am there not to judge but to help them. It became clear to me that overeating was often compensation for a temporary or lasting lack of satisfaction in my patients' lives. They found satisfaction in food knowing full well that this would make them fat.

My belief is that a person's relationship with their food, their self-image, and their weight as well as their self-esteem can be entirely explained by the structure of their primitive brain and how it operates.

In the oldest part of the brain is the hypothalamus. Its function is basic and essential: to ensure behavior that will guarantee our survival—to eat, fight, reproduce, and live and cooperate with others of our kind. To achieve this, the hypothalamus uses two small centers of extraordinary importance: one controlling reward and pleasure and the other punishment and discomfort. These structures appear in creatures as primitive as reptiles; hence it is sometimes called "the lizard brain." We share these primal urges with our cold-blooded neighbors; we all welcome and are drawn by pleasure, and do our best to avoid pain and discomfort.

The overweight person who uses a surfeit of food to neutralize discomfort or some suffering needs a strategy that connects displeasure into the circuit of pleasure.

Let me explain. When you try to lose weight and you make yourself do without that pleasurable moment of eating that makes your day a good one, you produce a negative or upsetting feeling. However, the following day when you get up and see that you have lost ½ pound or so, your body produces a pleasure response, you feel contentment. In fact, you are placing a layer of pleasure over a layer of displeasure. Hope is born, a wall of resistance forms between you and temptation, and there you are on your way.

However, to keep moving forward, you have to maintain this connection with pleasure. Ideally you should be able to tell someone about your progress, and this person will share your satisfaction. All it takes are words of congratulation to link yesterday's satisfaction with this morning's feelings of accomplishment and pleasure.

Only this kind of feedback loop can be given the name of close coaching, and only the Internet is capable of providing it to millions of people at the same time. This is the reason why I set up this coaching site on the Internet in France in May 2008, and it is my pride and joy. Since then I have established sites in six countries, and an online community of millions.

My Online Coaching in Practice

It All Starts with Calculating Your True Weight

When you reach the Dukan Diet website's home page (www.dukandiet .com), the first thing you will see is a True Weight calculator.

Your True Weight, as I have already said, is a weight that is both attainable and maintainable. I see too many patients chase after an unrealistically low weight, become frustrated, and abandon their efforts when they had in fact already achieved a perfectly "normal" weight. In fact there is no normal weight for everyone, but there is a normal weight for *you,* and that is *your* True Weight. How is it calculated?

1. *Age.* We put on weight with age. After age 20, each decade adds around a couple of pounds: 1.75 pounds if you are a woman, 2.6 pounds if you are a man.
2. *Gender.* Women do not tolerate weight gain as well as men, and I take this into account in my calculations.
3. *The most you have ever weighed in your life, apart from when pregnant.* Your body has a biological memory, and it remembers its highest weight.
4. *The least you weighed after age 20.* Between these two extreme

weights is what I call the "weight range." For example: if your maximum weight is 189 pounds and your minimum weight 128 pounds, the range is 61 pounds,

5. *The weight YOU would like to be at.* The more ambitious you are, even if deep down you are not sure that you could attain and maintain this "ideal" weight, the more you will rebel at the idea of a "sensible" weight.

6. *Your "cruise" weight.* This is the weight you have stayed at the longest during your life, a weight at which, or close to which, your body has long felt cozy and at which it likes to stay.

7. *Heredity.* Is its influence strong, average, or nonexistent? If there is a tendency in your family to put on weight, then it is best not to aim for an unrealistically low weight. You will only be fighting against forces mightier than yourself.

8. *The number of pregnancies.* Depending on the woman and the number of children, each child adds two pounds to the True Weight.

9. *The thickness of your skeleton.* A heavy skeleton adds x and a light one subtracts y from the sum.

Reaching Agreement About Your Target Weight

Next comes the moment when we compare our targets, the weight you would like to get down to and the True Weight I consider to be the weight you stand the best chance of attaining *and* maintaining.

Ideally both our targets will be the same or be very similar. However, quite often we do not agree.

Patients or website users seldom ask to weigh more than their True Weight. If you were to surprise me with this, I would be the first to applaud, as I know that you have the best chance of both attaining and, most of all, maintaining the right weight.

However, I never agree to supervise any weight loss that is not maintainable, because one of the chief factors why dieting fails to work is that people attempt to slim down to unrealistic levels. Usually my Internet patients trust me and go along with this weight. There are some who as they approach their target make a final attempt to get me to shift my position. Occasionally I agree to adjust their goal for a couple or a few more pounds while reexamining their progress.

Sometimes people have a confused mental image of their body. When this happens, losing weight will not turn a negative self-image into a positive one but will only exacerbate their issues when their efforts do not meet their ideal.

Outlining Your Treatment and Its Four Phases

When we agree on your target weight, you will receive the following proposal:

ATTACK PHASE

"If you decide to start today, day 1 of your treatment, you will start with an Attack phase that will last the right number of days for you and takes the weight to be lost and your specific features into account."

———————

Let's take the example of a 40-year-old woman, 5 foot 5 inches tall, who weighs 154 pounds, whose True Weight is 132 pounds, and who has therefore 22 pounds to lose. Adapting my program for her would mean a 4-day Attack phase and a loss of 4 pounds.

CRUISE PHASE

"Day 5 of your treatment, you will go into the second phase, the Cruise phase. How long this lasts depends on how much weight remains to be lost."

———————

Using the previous example, the Cruise phase should last 8 weeks. If this were you, at the end of 8 weeks you would have lost 22 pounds, and you would have gotten down to your True Weight on the date set when you subscribed.

Our site statistics for the first three years show that

- 70 percent of subscribers who are coached reach their True Weight on the date predicted on day 1.
- 25 percent get there, but with an average delay ranging from between 1 week and 3 months, depending on the difficulties encountered.
- 5 percent fail or disappear from sight without giving any explanation.

This is a success rate practically unmatched in the world of medical nutrition, especially given that two-thirds of these people had already followed more than four weight loss diets without any success at all.

CONSOLIDATION PHASE

The day after you achieve your True Weight, you receive the first e-mail for the new Consolidation Phase, which lasts 5 days for every pound lost.

Sticking with the example of a weight loss of 22 pounds, you will need 110 days to "consolidate" the weight you originally got down to.

From this moment onward, for the rest of your life, all you need concentrate your efforts on are three measures: protein Thursdays, giving up elevators and escalators, and eating 3 tablespoonfuls of oat bran per day.

PERMANENT STABILIZATION PHASE

The fourth phase, the Permanent Stabilization phase, starts the day after the Consolidation phase ends. It is designed to last for the rest of your life. And it's the stabilized weight that alone signals that an overweight person has been "cured" and can be removed from weight problems statistics.

Online stabilization begins once the Consolidation phase is at an end. It introduces twice-weekly monitoring, an e-mail with instructions for protein Thursdays, and a second e-mail on Mondays to manage the "six other days of freedom," What does it offer and how?

First of all, *my presence through the instructions and my daily, live personal chat sessions.*

Permanent supervision, watching to monitor any weight gain, and *a system of alerts* that enable us to take action as soon as a subscriber goes over the limit. Each time you have a 1 percentile weight gain, I send you out a new counterattack.

Let us consider the woman who lost 22 pounds. For her, each 2 pounds that she gains represents 1 percentile. Depending on how many percentiles are exceeded, she will require both more supervision and more encouragement to lose the additional weight. The aim is to get you to regain control as quickly as possible, because it is easier to lose weight you have just put on than it is to lose longer-established pounds.

Being Accepted and Signing Up

Once you know your True Weight and course of treatment, you can sign up at any time. As soon as you join, you will receive two extremely useful tools: your summary report and your "apartment." Let's start with the summary report.

Your Summary Report

In order for us to draw up this summary report, once you have signed up for coaching you will answer eighty questions that will allow us to see your weak points, your strong points, and the habits and behavior patterns responsible for your weight problem.

You receive back a confidential summary report of about twenty pages long. I would recommend that you show this to your doctor. This summary report helps you understand your situation better, and it gives me the means to show you how my method can be adapted to suit you, and you alone.

Your Apartment

Your "apartment" is a safe place with virtual rooms. Here you will find all the tools and structure you need to lose weight effectively:

- *Your digital fridge* containing the 100 foods for your Attack and Cruise phases: 72 proteins and 28 vegetables, with their nutritional values. A simple click, and you'll know all there is to know about the food you've chosen.
- *The store cupboard* contains 58 grocery products that accompany the diet, such as canned fish, smoked products, vinegars, mustards, teas, oat and wheat brans, sauces, spices, reduced-fat cocoa, corn flour. Take a look before you do your shopping.
- *Your dining room,* with a thick book on the table containing the 600 most popular recipes of our website users. If you are creative, send me your recipes and I'll reply in person with a small surprise gift.
- *Your lounge* with
  - Direct access to chat sessions so you can be with me for my in-person online chat sessions.
  - Your library, where you'll find all the major international weight loss books and methods, with a review of each one.
- *The gym* and its 20 videos, each one tackling a different muscle area: pectoral muscles, deltoids, stomach and buttock muscles, and so on. For extra body shaping, you can choose exercises from these videos to supplement your minimum compulsory program and the exercise instructions I send you every morning.
- *Your pharmacy* is in your bathroom cabinet. Here you'll find all the diet aids useful when trying to lose weight. They too come with a review to guide you, as there are thousands of different sorts over the world, and just how useful they are can vary enormously depending on their quality, effectiveness, and price.

Stimulating the Desire to Live Life to the Fullest

For a long time we have known that regular exercise releases endorphins, giving us pleasure from being physically active.

However, it has now been discovered that this action is infinitely more essential, as being active releases dopamine and serotonin, two neurotransmitters involved in the human brain's highest functions.

Dopamine increases the level of vital energy, motivation, feeling well, joy in being alive, and the desire to live life to the fullest, to plan projects and carry them out.

Serotonin supplies joy and pleasure in being alive.

Recent large-scale studies have shown that with serious depression, exercise was at least as effective as the most active antidepressants. This is especially important given that overweight people suffer from depression two to three times more frequently than the rest of the population.

The Coaching Service Itself

Again, what makes the coaching website and the service provided so completely innovative is that here you are treated as an individual by having a personalized relationship and dialogue. Furthermore, your progress is supported by our daily dialogue: your evening e-mail tells me how your day went, and I reply the following morning with my e-mail drawing up your daily instructions, which are adapted to your unique requirements.

My very first e-mail will present you with a panoramic view of your whole treatment, showing what happens in the four phases based on your personal situation.

In my second e-mail, I will set out your Attack Phase and the number of days you'll need to follow it.

As you go into the three other phases, I'll again send you an e-mail explaining their purpose and what you and I should expect from them.

From then onward, every morning, you'll receive your e-mail with instructions, written for you in reply to your report from the previous evening.

Your Evening Feedback Report Is Absolutely Vital

The information your evening feedback report provides me is my eyes and ears. Without it I cannot help you at all since I have *absolutely no way* of knowing what you did with my instructions. This report is short, and you can fill it out with only six clicks:

1. Your weight for the day.
2. Anything you may have eaten that you shouldn't have, graded according to a scale related to the food you lapsed with. You create this list just by clicking on ready-made categories, such as bread, cooked meats, cake, fats, alcohol, chocolate, and so on. Later on, if you don't understand why on a particular day your weight curve suddenly shot up when it was going down on a regular basis, all you need do is to click on your weight for that day, and the foods will be displayed that caused your odd gain.
3. Your motivation—you'll score this on a scale of 1 to 5, from euphoria to wanting to give up.
4. Your report of the exercise done.
5. Your degree of frustration on a scale of 1 to 5.
6. The food you have missed most in the day. When you start wanting the same food too much, I'll send you backup to help you keep going.

Decisions about you are taken based on these six parameters, and your instructions for the following morning can then be assembled and written. This is why I ask you not to forget about your evening report.

Your Daily Morning E-mail with Instructions

Your daily morning e-mail is my personal messenger and has three sections:

- Your eating instructions
- Your exercise instructions
- Motivational support

Your Eating Instructions

Your eating instructions will give you a wide choice of breakfasts, three lunches, and three dinners, a quick snack, and two menus—a more substantial one and a more elaborate one. If you don't fancy anything, you can always dip into the recipes on the website or try a dish again that you enjoyed before.

Your Exercise Instructions

Your exercise instructions will give you the compulsory program with walking to match your phase (20 minutes in the Attack phase, 30 minutes in the Cruise phase, 25 minutes in the Consolidation phase, and 20 minutes in the Permanent Stabilization phase), the four basic exercises, and the weight loss habits you need to follow.

There is also an optional program, which depends on how your treatment, your weight, and your habits are progressing.

Motivational Support

Every day you will receive motivational support as you get my feedback about how your previous day went and your weight, as well as my reactions to your lapses or self-control.

When everything is going well, I will tell you so. The satisfaction you give me I will share with you, and I will encourage you to keep going. Each step forward makes you want to take another, bigger step.

If you have had one or more lapses, you will have told me about it in the website column, which also grades them from the very minor to the very major. If you have succumbed, then the following morning, don't be surprised when I ask you to make up for this with a much stricter day and increased exercise.

Getting Through Stagnation

As most of my Internet patients progress, they experience a time of stagnation. This is when, having followed my instructions to the letter, their weight stubbornly refuses to budge. They may even—yes, this does happen—have gained a few ounces. If this happens to you, it is okay for 1, 2, or 3 days, but if you go for 5 or 6 days without results, things can get tricky, because you may wonder whether the stagnation is due to your body or to the method and be struck by a tremendous urge to comfort-eat.

This is when support is essential. Sometimes all it takes is a word of explanation to hold on for another day or two and allow the weight loss to finally appear on the scales. If you don't give up, it is the body's resistance that will finally give way. However, no one knows precisely when this will happen. The main thing is to hold on and not give in.

In difficult cases, it may become necessary to step up the pressure to force things along. I then might suggest a "blitz operation" with 3, 4, or even 5 days of Attack proteins with a much increased water intake, restricting salt, a full 60-minute walk, and an herbal detoxification agent. Then the stalled engine springs back into life.

My Daily Chat Session

Each day, I answer questions from subscribers live and in person. A number of female dietitians work alongside me to answer those general questions that are not addressed to me personally.

The questions cover every topic. There are lots about the foods you are allowed, as well as about "tolerated" foods. There are 30 or so foods in this category that do not officially belong on my authorized food list.

During my consultations, my answers during chat sessions, or my replies to e-mails, I sometimes agree to requests from individuals who would like to take the rough edges off their diet, as they have much weight to lose or because they are going through a very trying time emotionally. As long as this deviation from the prescribed diet prevented frustration and did not interfere with weight loss, I have given in to their friendly pressure.

For one person, it was adding a bit of cream cheese to an authorized oat bran pizza base. Another, a chocoholic, wanted a little fat-reduced cocoa. The same goes for light sour cream with "just 3 percent fat." And to improve the taste of muffins or the oat bran gingerbread (which can be found on my website), a small spoonful of cornmeal.

I call these foods "shock absorbers." However, they may only be used if your weight loss is on schedule and satisfactory. They have to be abandoned as soon as weight loss stagnates. Furthermore, we ration their use, both as far as quantity goes—for example, 1 teaspoonful of cocoa per day—as well as the number you can have—no more than 2 tolerated foods per day. You can find more information on www.dukandiet.com.

The dietitians who work alongside me during the chat sessions are all women who have lost weight with my method and who at times know it even better than I do. They are kind, understanding, and have great empathy and rapport. Sonya, Cristel, and Hannah look after the English speakers. Lorena and Mercedes look after the Spanish speakers.

Since the site was launched, I have already answered over 15,000 questions personally. Together these replies make up a body of information that more or less covers every scenario and every question that people might encounter during their treatment. You can access this information by using a search engine and typing in your keyword, such as "thyroid," for example, or "constipation," or "nonfat yogurt." You'll then see the 24 answers for thyroid or the 52 answers for constipation. Many subscribers simply dip into this store of information, finding everything they need here, and they read the daily chat session content to soak up what is happening within the community. The website is a mighty vessel with many different people on board, all sailing toward the same destination—to "be cured of being overweight."

———————

Dear reader, please understand that I have taken the time to go through this process with you as it is now an integral part of my method. Reading this book and applying its instructions are enough for you to lose weight and then permanently stabilize the weight you get down to. However, for anyone with a "complicated" weight or a long history of a "difficult condition" who has a genuine and serious need to lose weight but who does not feel confident about the battle looming before them, they will find the help and support they need in this.

INDEX

DUKAN DIET NATIONAL SURVEY ON SHORT-, MEDIUM-, AND LONG-TERM RESULTS

With the publication of this new edition of the Dukan Diet, I would like to ask a favor of my readers. The purpose of the questionnaire that follows is to collect as many replies as possible to enable us to set up the first weight study looking at more than 1,000 cases of weight loss greater than 17 pounds, which will help progress the science behind the Dukan Diet. In return we will keep you regularly informed of the progress of the study.

――――――――

Dear reader, only send me the completed questionnaire if you have definitely decided to follow this diet seriously, with the firm intention not only of losing weight but of stabilizing the weight by following the last two phases in my program, the Consolidation and the Permanent Stabilization phases.

As soon as we receive your first completed questionnaire, you will have started out with me on this diet, and I am convinced that this study will help you to follow it better. I will keep you informed about how this project is progressing, whose results will make a massive contribution to the fight against weight problems in the world. The study is going to be launched in nine languages and in seventeen countries at the same time. From its results, from you taking part, I hope to give my method—which will become yours too if it enables you to lose weight and conquer your weight problems—its final legitimacy and its reference value.

Please photocopy the questionnaire, fill it in, and send it to the address on page 279. If you are chosen to be part of the study, I will contact you.

- Your name and first name: . . . .
- Your postal address:

. . . .

City: . . . . State/Province . . . . . Zip/Postal Code . . . .

- E-mail address: . . . .
- Age: . . . .
- Gender: Male | Female
- Height in feet and inches . . . .
- Current weight (at the start of the diet): . . . .
- If you have started the Dukan Diet, how much weight have you already lost? . . . .
- Maximum weight ever weighed: . . . .
- Minimum weight ever weighed (after age 18): . . . .
- Number of diets already tried: . . . .
- Do you prefer? sweet | savory | no preference
- Do you need to eat big quantities? yes | no
- Do you snack between mealtimes? yes | no
- Does stress influence your weight? yes | no
- Do you have a family history of putting on weight? none | a little | average | a lot
- When you go on a diet, is losing weight: easy | difficult
- Do you walk for more than 20 minutes per day? yes | no
- Why do you want to lose weight? well-being | health | to be beautiful | to be seductive | to lead a normal life
- How did you come to read this book?

  A friend or colleague recommended it

  It was recommended in the press

Your doctor advised you to read it

Browsing in a bookshop

Through the Internet

Through a users forum (please specify): . . . .

Other (please specify): . . . .

If you have already lost weight using the Dukan Diet, I would be very grateful if you could let me know this by filling in this questionnaire and telling me how long ago you reached your True Weight and in particular if you carefully followed my program's two Consolidation and Permanent Stabilization phases.

If you supply your e-mail address, I will send you regular updates about this study. You will also be able to take part in chat room discussions to get replies to any questions that crop up as you follow this diet and for which the book does not provide the full answer.

To take part, please send your questionnaire to

Caradine

Dukan Diet National Study

6, rue Charles Fourier

75013 Paris

France

ABOUT THE AUTHOR

DR. PIERRE DUKAN has been a medical doctor specializing in human nutrition since 1973. He is the author of many works on nutrition for the scientific community, as well as works for the general public. He writes regularly in the press and appears on television. Dr. Dukan chairs R.I.P.O.S.T.E., an international association of nutritionists.

The popularity of Dr. Dukan's methods and works in countries as different in culture as Korea and Bulgaria show how he has become the most widely read French nutritionist in the world. In 2009, *The Dukan Method* was the best-selling book in Poland.

Nowadays, many health professionals and epidemiologists believe the Dukan Diet to be the method best equipped to put a halt to the weight problems that are still on the increase the world over.

Can't get enough of Dukan?

Discover the Complete Dukan Diet Library!

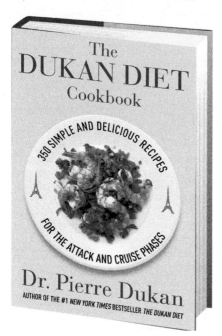

The Dukan Diet Cookbook has 350 delicious recipes to help make losing weight a pleasure!

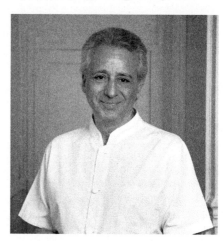

25% **Discount** on Our Personalized Diet Coaching

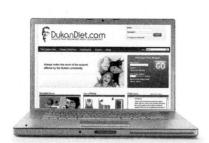

Visit www.dukandiet.com and enter code: **CAD25**

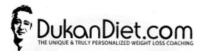

The Dukan Diet products you need to succeed!

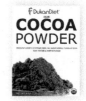

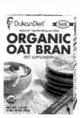

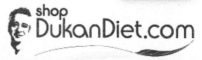